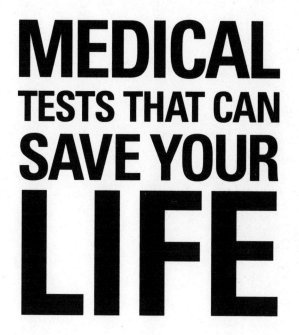

MEDICAL
TESTS THAT CAN
SAVE YOUR
LIFE

MEDICAL
TESTS THAT CAN
SAVE YOUR
LIFE

21 TESTS YOUR DOCTOR WON'T ORDER...
UNLESS YOU KNOW TO ASK

David Johnson, Ph.D., and David Sandmire, M.D.

with Daniel Klein

RODALE

Notice
This book is intended as a reference volume only, not as a medical manual. The information given here is designed to help you make informed decisions about your health. It is not intended as a substitute for any treatment that may have been prescribed by your doctor. If you suspect that you have a medical problem, we urge you to seek competent medical help.

Mention of specific companies, organizations, or authorities in this book does not imply endorsement by the publisher, nor does mention of specific companies, organizations, or authorities imply that they endorse this book.

Internet addresses and telephone numbers given in this book were accurate at the time it went to press.

Printed in the United States of America

Book design by Leanne Coppola/Abbate Design

Library of Congress Cataloging-in-Publication Data

Johnson, David W. (David Wayne), date.
    Medical tests that can save your life : 21 tests your doctor won't order . . . unless you know to ask / David Johnson and David Sandmire, with Daniel Klein.
        p.   cm.
    Includes index.
    ISBN 1–57954–732–X paperback
    1. Diagnosis.   2. Medicine, Popular.   I. Sandmire, David.   II. Klein, Daniel M.
III. Title.
RC71.J64 2004
616.07'5—dc22   2004007790

Distributed to the book trade by St. Martin's Press

2   4   6   8   10   9   7   5   3   1   paperback

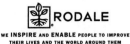

CONTENTS

PART THREE: THE TESTS

PREFACE

This book has the potential to save your life.

In it, we'll describe 21 medical tests that can detect deadly diseases when they're in their earliest stages, and thus are still treatable. We'll tell you how to figure out which tests to have, and where and when to have them. The medical environment can be a confusing, frightening, and downright frustrating place. This book can help with much of that.

In Part One, we'll explain how the world of medical testing got to be so difficult. In order to figure out whether or not you should have certain tests, you'll compile a personal risk profile that includes your medical history, your family's medical history, your social history (Do you smoke? Drink? Work in a dangerous environment?), and more. In the next chapter, we'll walk you through these questions and give you a worksheet to fill out, and in the following chapter, we'll explain how to get what you need from your doctor and insurer, and what to do if they're not cooperative.

Part Two of this book is organized by diseases and conditions. They're listed alphabetically to make it easier for you to find the information you're seeking. You'll want to read each of the chapters, however, to determine your risk level for each condition. It's important for you to remember, as you read, that many people are at high risk for diseases and don't even know it!

In each chapter, we define the condition and walk you through determining your own risk level. We then let you know what tests to request from your doctor.

Part Three describes each of the tests in detail. So, once you decide which test to have, you'll get a good idea of what is involved in the process (how long it takes, what actually happens), the reliability of the test, the health risks involved in taking the test (if any), and the cost of the test. Lastly, we'll list available treatments if your test results happen to be positive. Those treatments are addressed in an appendix in the back of the book.

Disease prevention is ultimately your job, not your doctor's. Armed with the knowledge this book provides, you will be able to walk into your next checkup with a list of medical tests that you want to have. Best of all, you—the well-informed patient—will be able to tell your doctor exactly why.

ONE

USING
THIS BOOK

INTRODUCTION

A forty-year-old Irish-American man goes to his family doctor for his annual check-up. The nurse dutifully weighs him and takes his pulse and blood pressure (all normal). The doctor asks him how he has been feeling ("Fine, thanks"); listens to his heart and lungs for abnormal sounds (none); feels his abdomen for masses or enlarged liver or spleen (none); examines his testicles for masses and checks him for hernia (no problems); looks at his skin for abnormal growths (none); examines his ears, eyes, and throat for lesions (none); and examines lymph nodes in his neck, armpit, and groin for enlargement (all okay). Then the nurse returns to take blood samples for a lipid profile (total cholesterol, with HDL, LDL, and triglycerides) and a hematocrit—a blood test that checks blood count (all come back well within the normal range).

When the doctor phones after the test results are in, he tells the man that he should try to lose a few pounds—but other than that, he's in perfect health.

Eight months later, the man suffers a major heart attack that kills him.

We have all heard variations on this story. And our usual

reaction is a resigned, "That's fate for you," or "It just goes to prove there's only so much a doctor can tell you."

Wrong. The doctor could have told the man in our story a great deal more if he had ordered a simple and inexpensive test known as the percent transferrin saturation test. The results of that test would have revealed that this man had an abnormally high amount of iron in his body—a serious risk factor for coronary heart disease (CHD). The doctor could have then put the man on an iron-restricted diet and on a regimen of removing a pint of blood from his system every 2 weeks until his iron load was back to normal. Had the doctor done this test and prescribed that treatment, it is highly unlikely that this heart attack would have ever occurred. In short, the test would have saved the man's life.

But why hadn't this doctor ordered a percent transferrin saturation test? He certainly wasn't incompetent by today's standards. In fact, he was performing his duties precisely according to prevailing medical doctrine: Only order an "unusual" test if there are symptoms of a particular disease.

Well, the man in question certainly did not display any symptoms of CHD, or any other disease, for that matter. And the transferrin saturation test *is* unusual, since a relatively small percentage of people have the life-threatening condition of iron overload.

Regardless, there was strong indirect evidence that this particular man was at risk for iron overload. First, there was his family history: His father and siblings had all developed CHD at an early age although they did not have the usual risk factors of elevated blood pressure or elevated cholesterol or triglyceride levels. So it was highly likely that something else accounted for the high preponderance of CHD in this family. Iron overload was one of several possible candidates for that role. Second, this man ran a much higher than average possibility of having hereditary hemochromatosis—a genetic disorder that causes abnormally high absorption of iron from food—simply by dint of the fact that he was of

Irish descent. The Irish happen to be much more likely to inherit this disorder than other European peoples.

Given these two salient facts, the doctor certainly should have ordered the percent transferrin saturation test. For this particular man coming in for a routine check-up, this lifesaving test should have been done.

There are a significant number of medical tests that doctors rarely order. But given specific circumstances, these tests should be routine for certain patients. Every one of these tests has the potential to save your life.

The Medical Mind-Set

We wish we could say that the doctor in the above scenario is atypical, but he is not. Not at all.

According to a recent study, one in three doctors withholds information from his patients that could benefit them. In particular, this means that these doctors may not tell their patients about screening tests that could detect potentially fatal diseases in early, treatable stages. The reason? These tests and procedures are not covered by the patient's medical insurance.

Many lifesaving medical tests are expensive, so medical insurers and HMOs usually won't pay for them unless the doctor observes active symptoms of a disease (or he is tracking the progress of a disease that is already diagnosed). Doctors often will not recommend a test that isn't covered, because they don't want to be stuck with the cost if the patient can't pay for it.

The doctor in the above scenario did not look deeply into his patient's family medical history or into the possible genetic risks for another fundamental reason: This doctor had the same medical mind-set as the great majority of physicians and was only looking for active symptoms of diseases. For the most part, he was not looking for the predictors of future diseases.

BUYER BEWARE: FULL-BODY CT SCAN

You may be familiar with some of the tests we describe here, but the one predictive test you have undoubtedly heard of is the much-advertised full-body CT scan. Currently, these scans are all the rage with what some wags have termed "the worried wealthy." With a price tag between $900 and $1,400 (so far, insurance companies refuse to reimburse for it), this procedure is being offered by clinics and private mobile screening companies to everyone—regardless of whether or not they have any risk factors. The full-body CT scan is exactly what it says it is: a visualization of most of your interior anatomy. It promises to catch just about any detectable disease—particularly cancer—in its earliest stages.

Although we strongly recommend tests that can lead to early detection and early treatment of a disease, we do not endorse the full-body CT scan for everybody. Rather, we believe that your health, time, and pocketbook are far better served by getting the specific medical test tailored to your personal health risks.

It is far more effective and less hazardous to identify your risks for a disease and then pinpoint precisely which tests are most relevant to your profile. It makes much more sense to go

Early Detection Medicine Comes of Age

Most of us grew up regarding the family doctor as all-knowing and all-caring. We never doubted for a moment that the man in the white coat held our interest—and our health—paramount to any other considerations.

We now have to revise our thinking. The explosion of new medical discoveries, including new screening and treatment options, has made it increasingly difficult for doctors to keep up-

directly to the screening tests that apply to you, for example, to get the transvaginal ultrasound for ovarian cancer if you are at particularly high risk for developing that disease, or the abdominal ultrasound for renal cell carcinoma, the spiral CT scan for lung cancer, or the ERCP for pancreatic cancer. In this way, the chances of the benefits outweighing the risks are likely to be much higher than taking the shotgun approach of a full-body CT scan. In the population as a whole, the chances of stumbling upon an early cancer in some organ system are literally one in a thousand—not very common!

We cannot endorse the full-body scan for everyone for another reason: Research suggests that the amount of radiation received in these scans is likely to be more dangerous than patients are led to believe. Furthermore, a full-body CT scan often detects small tumors that are not cancerous—doctors wryly refer to these as "incidentalomas." The appearance of these harmless masses often leads to unnecessary further testing, additional risk, and great expense—not to mention great anxiety for patients while they wait for results that are negative a great deal of the time.

to-date on the best way to approach an individual patient. Also, health care plans have hamstrung physicians—limiting the new tests and treatments they can "afford" to offer to their patients. Together, these trends mean that all too often, you are not getting the full story about your health or treatment options. And there is only one solution: You must become the best-informed patient that you can possibly be.

For centuries, medicine has operated with two goals: to prevent injury and illness and to cure an existing illness or injury. But because of new technology, medicine has a new goal: to detect illness at an early stage and to treat it before it becomes debilitating and incurable.

The current possibilities for early diagnosis and effective early treatment are positively revolutionary. Yet early detection and early treatment medicine is possibly the most underutilized piece of medicine today—by both health care providers and health care consumers alike.

Just how did we end up not taking full advantage of this incredible medical opportunity?

The full explanation is a complex story of conflicting economic, political, social, and professional agendas, not to mention a good portion of ignorance and psychological resistance. Medical testing can be expensive, invasive, or just plain embarrassing. Due to the state of health care in this country, you may find it difficult to get your doctor to order a test and even more difficult to get your insurer to pay. But as you'll learn, the hassle is well worth it. It can save your life.

Health Care Economics

High on the list of reasons for the underuse of medical testing is basic economics: Many of these procedures are expensive. We do not want to spend money on a medical procedure that, in all likelihood, will show that we are not sick. However, this attitude often proves to be a false economy, since addressing a disease in its early stages is almost always far less expensive than treating an advanced disease. But to a patient with no symptoms and a family to support, springing for a $400 MRI seems like a reckless expenditure.

And if it seems that way to the patient, you can bet the farm that it will feel that way to the insurance company. In many cases, this, too, is short-term thinking: Insurance companies and government agencies end up paying more for a cure for an advanced dis-

X-RAYS

X-rays were discovered in 1895, but most x-raying done prior to World War I was available only in the largest hospitals and medical schools. The expenses of x-ray machines made for tough decisions about which patients would benefit most from this remarkable new diagnostic tool.

By the time radiology became a hospital-based specialty in the 1930s, major turf wars between doctors and hospitals had broken out. Suddenly, radiology was a big-buck enterprise. But there were no national standards for answering the basic economic questions: Who would own the x-ray equipment? How would the fees be divided between physicians and hospitals? And most important, who would be x-rayed and who would not?

ease than they would have had to pay for the early-detection test plus the early medical care.

In recent years, the cost of early detection tests has risen for a number of reasons, but the main reason the cost of these tests has risen so much is that the rising tide of all medical costs has lifted the diagnostic tests boat.

RISING MEDICAL COSTS

Our current health care system's reimbursement scheme for diagnostic medical tests represents a compromise between two opposing philosophies. One viewpoint is that the government should provide universal health care coverage to all Americans (sometimes referred to as "compulsory health insurance" or "socialized medicine"). The other view is that our health care system should mirror our capitalist economic framework—that is, the marketplace should provide multiple, competing health care systems so that only the most efficient and cost-effective health care delivery programs survive. Unfortunately, it's apparent that compromising hasn't done much to reduce medical costs.

MEDICARE AND MEDICAID

In 1965, President Lyndon B. Johnson signed legislation that established health insurance for social security beneficiaries (Medicare) and grants to states to provide care for the poor and indigent (Medicaid). With guaranteed reimbursement for medical tests and services, physicians and hospitals had little incentive to be frugal. Medicare quickly became the goose that laid the golden egg for physicians. As historian Ronald Numbers noted, the rate of increase in physician fees more than doubled in the first year following passage of Medicare. Medicare opened the floodgates for physicians to overutilize medical tests, which were becoming a major income-generator for physicians.

Medicare funds received by the nation's hospitals doubled between 1970 and 1975, and then doubled again by 1980. Even after controlling for general inflation, the average cost of a day's stay in the hospital more than doubled between 1966 and 1976. Hospital and physician fees began to spiral out of control.

Though Medicare and Medicaid were designed to improve public access to vital medical tests and other services, they set into motion a rate of medical fee inflation that made health care more expensive than it had ever been.

HMOs

Believing that efficiency and price controls could be attained most effectively through free market competition, Richard Nixon signed the HMO Act of 1973. Since physicians and hospitals were pre-paid at a fixed rate, there would be no financial incentive for the overuse of medical tests and other expensive procedures. Instead, HMOs would be rewarded for ordering fewer, rather than more, medical tests.

As one physician drolly put it, "The problem with incentives is that they work." If a physician and a hospital know ahead of time that they will receive a set amount of money for a patient of a particular disease category, regardless of how they care for that patient, they stand to make more money by ordering fewer diagnostic tests.

And it can become even more insidious than that. David Himmelstein, M.D., associate professor at Harvard Medical School, reported to *Time* magazine that he was booted out of a particular HMO because he refused to abide by the HMO's "gag rule"—a rule that did not allow him to tell a patient that there was a possibly more effective, but definitely more expensive treatment for her condition than the one allowed by the HMO. Further, Himmelstein stated that some HMOs offered doctors steep financial incentives (what he referred to as bribes) to minimize costs. It's a no-brainer: As long as a physician is put in this situation, there is a possibility that patients will receive inadequate care.

MALPRACTICE SUITS

In addition to Medicare and Medicaid, there was another major stimulus for the overuse of diagnostic medical tests: American patients began to sue their doctors more frequently. Thus, a doctor would order a test—even if he thought there would be a 98 percent chance of it being negative—because he suspected that the patient would sue if he turned out to be wrong.

This liability crisis has grown to incredible proportions in recent years, forcing the cost of malpractice insurance premiums to skyrocket, which, in turn, causes all medical costs to the consumer to increase. But perhaps the most destructive consequence of this crisis is the rupture in the relationship between doctors and their patients. Not only are patients mistrustful of their doctors, but the fear of a devastating malpractice suit has also made doctors mistrustful of their patients. In this atmosphere, doctor and patient become adversaries rather than partners in maintaining the patient's health.

Now, the patients aren't the only ones frustrated by the system. Physicians are largely unhappy with it as well, particularly older physicians who recall earlier days when they had greater autonomy and self-determination. In this new century, physicians are bogged down in bureaucracy. To make matters worse, large employers

A PROMISING NEW ECONOMIC TREND IN EARLY DETECTION MEDICINE

Faced with a "medical industrial complex" that is outrageously expensive and is nerve-wracking to navigate, many Americans have looked to independent, mobile medical testing units as a way to receive diagnostic tests without the middleman. The largest of these companies is Life Line Screening, formed in 1993 and operating in 33 states around the nation. By operating in high volume and offering a very limited set of screening examinations, independent screening companies like Life Line are able to significantly reduce the costs of these procedures. Life Line focuses on screening for the early signs of illnesses that are common in the general population, that come on quickly with few preliminary warning signs, and that, if detected, can be treated successfully. Since Medicare and most other third-party payers of medical bills refuse to authorize many screening medical tests in symptomless patients without risk factors, Life Line offers an inexpensive alternative to wading through the quicksand of the medical industrial complex.

have become the principal customers of managed care, placing one more obstacle between the physician and patient. In this arrangement, the patients are told which physicians they can see, and the physicians are told which services they can provide.

The Big Loser: Early Detection/ Early Treatment Medicine

The unhappy implications for early detection/early treatment medicine are obvious: Since physicians are told which patients qualify for expensive diagnostic tests, many patients who could benefit

The advantage of independent screening companies is that a physician referral is not required. Thus, for $35, you can have a Carotid Doppler Ultrasound examination to assess your risk of developing a stroke, the results of which are reviewed by board-certified radiologists and vascular surgeons—a procedure and evaluation that would cost between $300 and $500 if performed in the hospital! Life Line offers inexpensive screening for abdominal aortic aneurysm (weakening and bulging out of the large artery in the abdomen), peripheral vascular disease (blockage of arteries supplying blood to the legs), and osteoporosis. In each case, the actual procedure is inexpensive (typically about $35), noninvasive (that is, very little risk associated with the test), and has the potential for detecting "silent killers." In a one-stop shopping package, you can be screened for strokes, atherosclerosis, aneurysms, and osteoporosis for the grand total of $120 without the need for a physician referral.

from a particular diagnostic test are denied access to it. Instead, the doctor is only directed by guidelines for the general population. For example, it is the rare asymptomatic patient who benefits from an MRI of the carotid artery, so it is considered inefficient to order this test for a patient who displays no symptoms.

The insurance companies look at it this way: If only 5 percent of the asymptomatic population benefits from a particular diagnostic test, it makes better financial sense not to pay for this test. They can then pay for the medical costs if and when patients show symptoms of this disease—say, after they actually have a stroke! This approach is the inevitable outcome of our shrinking health care dollar. Its pragmatic philosophy of "the greatest good for the greatest number of patients" is admirable, but the individual can too easily end up short-changed in the process.

In the current situation, physicians do not have incentive to compile an exhaustive record of a patient's complete medical history, her complete genetic make-up, and a detailed survey of her living environment and her lifestyle practices. Thus, they cannot calculate her complete disease-risk profile and determine if she could benefit from a diagnostic procedure. Because the doctor is only following guidelines for the general population, he falls back on his old tried-and-true method of operation: He only orders a particular test if an overt symptom is present.

In the midst of this mess, we, as patients, must keep our heads clear and our backbones straight. We cannot become our own doctors, but we can become the next best thing: thoroughly informed patients who insist on the best possible medical options available. And it all begins with an understanding of how to compile your own personal risk profile.

YOUR PERSONAL RISK PROFILE

In order to decide whether or not you should have a particular diagnostic test, you should know your personal risk profile. Your profile is a compilation of risk factors that apply specifically to you: your own health and its history, your genetic make-up, your extended family's medical history, your lifestyle and habits, and your living and working environment.

Precisely how to weigh each particular risk factor in your profile is an inexact science. Some risk factors send up more red flags than others. But one general rule plainly applies to all risk factors and the decision of whether or not they warrant a diagnostic test: The more risk factors you have, the greater your overall risk.

In Parts Two and Three, we'll describe diseases and their corresponding risk factors. It makes good sense to have your personal risk profile already compiled and assembled before you review those chapters, so that you can determine their relevance to you as efficiently and accurately as possible. More important, you should have your personal risk profile neatly filled out and ready to go for that moment when you pop it on your doctor's desk.

We've included a personal risk worksheet that you may want

(continued on page 18)

Age

Gender

Medical History

Racial or Ethnic Background

Family Medical History

  First-Degree Relatives

     Parents

     Siblings

     Children

  Second-Degree Relatives

     Grandparents

     Aunts and Uncles

     Cousins

Social History

    Smoking History

    Alcohol Use

    Diet

    Exercise

Environmental Risk Factors

to photocopy and complete as you go through this chapter. You'll
want to keep track of your risk profile and write it down.

Age and Gender

When your doctor (with the ever-present, over-the-shoulder guidance
of your insurer) determines whether or not you are a candidate for
a particular diagnostic test, he will probably consider your age and
gender to be critical risk factors. If you are a male over 50, he will
probably order an annual PSA test to determine if you have signs of
prostate cancer. Or, if you are a female, he will probably recommend
an annual Pap smear 3 years after becoming sexually active, or after
reaching age 21 to determine if you have signs of cervical cancer.

Personal Medical History

Most of us have a fairly good idea of what diseases and treatments
we have had during the course of our lives, but critical details may
escape us. For example, you may know that you had rheumatic
fever when you were six, but not know for how long you were sick,
what exact treatments you received, and most important, what
residual effects of the disease—like a heart murmur—remained
after the disease and treatment had run their course. Further, you
may not have ever been fully informed about what diseases you
once had, particularly those you had as a child.

There are two basic sources for this information: your parents
and your doctors. Be sure to ask your parents or other surviving
relatives about your personal medical history when you sit down
to record your family medical history.

Your doctors, present and past, should have detailed medical
files on your medical history. You are entitled to copies of these files!
Some doctors may resist turning them over to you, arguing that you
are incapable of interpreting the technical information properly and

accurately. More likely, the doctor may argue that copying this information is too burdensome and costly for his staff. An offer to pay the costs of reproducing the files may ease the way, but there is absolutely no reason to be cowed into taking "No" for an answer.

These files may be voluminous, hard to decipher, and very poorly organized, so be prepared for long evenings of wading through them. Further, you will probably need a medical dictionary, a medical encyclopedia, and a *Physician's Desk Reference* (for identifying medications) on hand in order to make sense of much of this material. Using the Internet can also be quite helpful. It's a little like going back to school—not entirely a lot of fun, but well worth it. And you may be surprised and find it more interesting and enlightening than you would have guessed.

Your goal in this process is to come up with a brief but exhaustive list of your medical history: diseases incurred, their duration, treatment, and residual effects; and the diagnostic tests you have already had, particularly those that have not been appropriately followed up.

Genetic Makeup

Your racial and ethnic background is a part of your family medical history, but it is helpful to consider it separately when assembling your risk profile. Some racial and ethnic groups are more at risk for certain diseases than others. Like age and gender, your ethnic makeup can help pinpoint your risk, but unlike age and gender, ethnicity is often not a consideration of your doctor when he calculates your risk. The solution once again: Figure it out yourself.

Of course, most Americans are racial and ethnic salads, an Irishman in the family tree here, a German there, an Asian or mid-Easterner over there. It is not always easy to figure out just how "diluted" a particular genetic proclivity is if, say, you have only one Irish grandfather. Nonetheless, your ethnic make-up should be figured into your overall risk profile as one more factor that can help you make a decision about a particular test.

Extended Family Medical History

Clearly, a critical component of your risk profile is your family medical history. Since many diseases have a genetic basis, it is important to know about the specific types of health problems that your family members have experienced. Your physician will primarily be interested in the health (illnesses and cause of death) of your first-degree relatives—your parents, siblings, and children. But although somewhat less important, the health history of your second-degree relatives—grandparents, aunts, uncles, and cousins—should be tabulated as well.

Physicians John Coulehan, M.D., and Marian Block, M.D., have compiled the categories of illness that comprise a complete family medical history. You'll want to take note of each of them on your personal risk worksheet.

1. **Clear-cut hereditary diseases:** These are conditions caused by single genes with very predictable patterns of inheritance, for example, cystic fibrosis, sickle-cell anemia, Huntington's disease, or muscular dystrophies.

2. **Family diseases:** These are conditions in which multiple genetic and environmental factors play a significant role and whose presence in your family history raises your risk of developing a particular disease. But unlike clear-cut hereditary diseases, the patterns of inheritance are not as obvious. Good examples of such familial diseases are type 2 diabetes, coronary artery disease, breast cancer, and alcoholism.

3. **Family traits:** These are characteristics (as compared to diseases) that run in families, such as obesity and short stature.

THE ETIQUETTE OF GATHERING YOUR FAMILY HEALTH HISTORY

Getting all of your family members to contribute to your family health history can be a dicey business. There is often a family member who responds point-blank that his health history is "none of your business," not to mention the family member who simply does not have time for such "nonsense." In both cases, these will probably be family members who are of the "ignorance-is-bliss" school about their own personal health risks.

One simple strategy for dealing with this problem is to work around these recalcitrant family members by getting the relevant health information about them from other relatives. Mothers are often the best resource here.

But another strategy is to convince your family members that it is a two-way street, that you will share with them your own health history and those of the relatives you have in common, thus giving them an opportunity to construct their own family health history and risk profile. And you will do most of the work, which is always a strong argument!

Finally, some people have discovered that they can make gathering the family health history one part of a larger, less threatening, and more sentimental enterprise: writing your family's general family history, including the relocations, adventures, jobs, people, and places in your family. The older members of your family will likely be attracted to such a project and may more readily add health issues to the overall story.

4. **Family illnesses as environmental risk factors:** If members of your immediate family suffer from disorders like autism or depression, there may be nongenetic effects on your own health, particularly psychological effects.

5. **Family infectious diseases and toxic exposures:** Clearly, if a member of your immediate family suffers from an infectious disease, like hepatitis A, you will be at a much greater than average risk for contracting this disease than the general population.

   Similarly, if members of your immediate family suffer or have suffered from environmental diseases such as lead poisoning or pneumoconiosis (black lung disease, caused by airborne particles) you will be at greater risk of developing the same diseases if you've lived or worked in the same environment.

Your Social History

Social history is a collective term that describes your lifestyle and habits (for example, smoking and use of alcohol and recreational drugs), diet, level of exercise, living environment, occupational environment, and sexual history (particularly your possible exposure to sexually transmitted diseases.) Each of these components can profoundly impact your risk for getting a particular disease, and therefore each belongs in your overall risk assessment.

CIGARETTE SMOKING

Obviously, cigarette smoking is the source of much illness and suffering, increasing your likelihood of emphysema; chronic bronchitis; heart disease; and cancers of the mouth, pharynx, esophagus, lung, and bladder. For most of these illnesses, the severity of the risk is proportional to the number of "pack-years" you've smoked—that is, the number of packs of cigarettes per day times the number of years you've smoked that amount. So if you've smoked two packs per day for 15 years, you have a 30 pack-year smoking history.

ALCOHOL ABUSE

Although the health benefits of one or two glasses of wine per day are currently being touted in the medical press, alcohol abuse can be devastating to one's health. Chronic abuse of alcohol is associated with peripheral nerve disease and Korsakoff's syndrome, a form of amnesia. It is implicated as well in inflammation of the esophagus, stomach, liver, and pancreas. Excessive alcohol consumption is also associated with liver cirrhosis; hypertension; poor blood-clotting ability; and cancers of the head, neck, esophagus, stomach, liver, pancreas, and breast.

DIET

Your dietary habits are another important component of your social history. Excessive calorie intake can lead to obesity, which is a risk factor for several diseases, including heart disease and Type 2 diabetes. A diet rich in cholesterol and saturated fats may make you more likely to suffer a heart attack, stroke, or peripheral vascular disease. Poorly balanced diets can lead to several different types of vitamin or mineral deficiencies. A deficiency of calcium in the diet, for example, can increase your risk for osteoporosis.

EXERCISE

Information about exercise and activity level is valuable to one's risk profile. Lack of exercise can contribute to osteoporosis, obesity, and cardiovascular disease. On the other hand, excessive exercise or activity may predispose you to injury, for example, shin splints and stress fractures in runners, knee injuries in football players and skiers, and carpal tunnel syndrome in painters and keyboard operators.

ENVIRONMENTAL HEALTH RISKS

The air (and dust) you breathe, the water you drink, the amount and quality of sun rays you are exposed to, the plants and animals you are in regular contact with, and the chemicals and metals in your living environment all may constitute health hazards. They should all be calculated into your personal risk profile.

You can determine your regional environmental health risks by requesting a complete report of the status of your living environment from the Environmental Protection Agency or from local environmental organizations. When doing this, be sure to ask for a historical overview of environmental risks in your area, including any industries that may have been there in the past.

Many of your home environment health risks can be determined by a thorough cataloguing of the chemicals you have in your house, such as those in cleaning materials and paint and repair materials.

GETTING WHAT YOU NEED
FROM YOUR DOCTOR

Okay, you have your personal risk profile together, and after reading this book, you'll have made a list of the tests you want. What now?

Well, for some of these tests, one option is to simply go to an independent medical testing unit and get the test and its results without bothering with the middlemen—your personal doctor and your third party payer. There's nothing wrong with that, especially since the price is right.

But not all early-detection tests are available through these independent units. If you cannot get the ones you believe are appropriate, you'll have to go through your own doctor. How do you get your doctor to take you seriously? In the absolute best-case scenario, you will be able to convince him to order the test *and* to plead your case to your insurer to get them to pay. This is not often an easy task, to say the least.

Doctor Knows Best, Right?

There is another reason why you may want to consult with your doctor before ordering a test: because you value his advice.

This may seem like an old-fashioned, sentimental concept. But, of course, your doctor is ideally the best resource you have for discussing your health. These days, you will have to make sure that your doctor schedules enough time with you to discuss test options thoroughly. And you will have to be confident that he is willing to listen to you and even learn a thing or two—like the details of your particular risk profile.

But it's important to remember that, when it comes to diagnostic testing, your doctor may not know best.

Physicians practice their art the way it was taught to them during their formal training. Doctors are trained to diagnose disease and then prescribe the proper treatment, so most of them use medical tests for only this purpose. Your doctor may also have trouble reconciling what is best for you with what is permitted by your HMO or insurer. With cost control utmost in mind, the HMO decides which tests will be paid for and also determines the criteria for a patient to have the test. Doctors are essentially employees of these HMOs—if they don't play by the company rules, they can be removed from it.

But wait one minute—shouldn't *you* be the one to decide?

Getting Your Doctor on Your Side

The first step to having an intelligent discussion with your doctor is seeing the situation from his point of view. So, start by putting on a white coat and looking frazzled. Just kidding . . . sort of.

Doctors *are* frazzled much of the time. Their work is demanding. Almost every decision and diagnosis they make can have momentous consequences—in some cases, life or death consequences. This, alone, can cause serious stress. But then add to that an excessive workload and voluminous paperwork, much of it coming from HMOs, insurers, and government agencies. And then put all of this into the context of a practice whose independence is limited by HMO restrictions and that is constantly in danger of malpractice lawsuits. Some serious frazzlement is bound to ensue.

And that is only one half of the equation. A doctor spends the whole day with patients—people who usually come into the office in a state of fear and anxiety. Plus, of course, these people are often sick, which may not bring out the most appealing parts of their personalities. In short, a doctor sees people day in and day out who are often desperate and impatient for help and relief. It would be difficult for even the best of us to be unerringly cheerful and unhurried with this kind of work life.

In order to have the best discussion possible about diagnostic tests, you should understand one particular thing: When physicians are surveyed about which characteristics make for the most "difficult" patients, they frequently cite patients who have a negative, critical, and suspicious attitude toward health care in general.

Well, that could describe many of us. Truth to tell, you may be looking into diagnostic tests on your own because you don't trust your doctor to do it for you. But it would be in your best interest to keep the attitude under wraps as much as possible when you initiate a discussion with your physician about medical testing.

Getting Your Physician to Listen to You

Getting your physician to listen to you begins before you even set foot in his office. It starts when you make your appointment.

Be very clear with your doctor's appointments assistant about the exact nature of your visit. This is not a routine checkup. You are not coming in with a symptom or disease complaint. No, you want to have a thorough consultation about diagnostic tests that you believe you should take.

Further, you must say that you believe that this will take more time than the standard allotment of 20 minutes for a checkup. Most doctors' schedules do not allow for extended conversations. A hurried discussion leads to the possibility of misunderstanding, and your misunderstanding of the efficacy of a medical test or the success rate of a medical procedure may breed false expectations. Similarly, your physician's misunderstanding about your personal risks and concerns may limit his ability to effectively address them.

"So please, Appointments Secretary, schedule this consultation for a time when the doctor is under the fewest time constraints." For most physicians, this usually means the first or last appointment of the day.

Now, it is no secret that appointments secretaries are often abrupt, even uncompromising. They are not used to patients who request any conditions on their visits. We can only suggest that you be cordial, but be firm. You are the consumer, after all, as hard as that may be to remember. For one thing, as the consumer, you do have the option of changing doctors if you do not get what you want—see page 31 for more information.

One way to make this exchange easier is to say up front that you are not in any hurry, that you want to see the doctor for this consultation when it is most convenient for him. This is not a line that most appointments secretaries hear often, and hearing it may reduce their own stress.

Okay, Now We Arrive at the Consultation Itself

First, come to the consultation as well-informed as possible. The more knowledgeable you are about a particular medical test and about your personal risk profile, the more time your physician will take listening to your argument for that test.

Printed matter helps immeasurably in this regard. For example, bring along articles, books, and printouts from respectable medical Web sites about the diagnostic tests that you want him to consider. Bookmark and highlight the parts of this material most relevant to your case—for example, a section on an unusual subgroup (Children of two parents who died of stroke? Irishmen? People who live near battery manufacturing plants?) that is at heightened risk for a disease you want to be tested for.

Also bring along your own personal risk profile, highlighting the sections relevant to the disease in question. You may want to spend the time to type up your risk profile just for this disease on a single piece of paper telling exactly why you, personally, have an usually high risk for this disease and therefore should be tested for it.

Your doctor may not express it, but we guarantee he will be impressed—impressed enough to take you seriously. Doctors very quickly gauge their patients' level of understanding of a medical problem and adjust their communication accordingly. If, right off the bat, a patient demonstrates solid knowledge, the doctor is more likely to respond with in-depth and informative answers. Contrarily, when a patient does not do her homework prior to the appointment, the doctor is likely to skip the hard parts and cut to the chase with a quick and dirty explanation that leaves the patient with an incomplete understanding.

Remember, aside from the nagging business of HMO accountants, your doctor may be skeptical of your arguments for genuine medical reasons. In many cases, there is no clear medical consensus on testing. When a clinical course of action is not so clear-cut, it is more likely that physician and patient will disagree about how to proceed. But it is in these "gray zones" that your physician should be more open to your opinion, particularly if it is an informed opinion.

You should also spend some time considering your personal approach to the discussion. You are essentially on a sales mission and therefore should avail yourself of all the sales techniques you can muster. Charm, for example, often works beautifully.

The fact that your doctor may perceive himself as a potential target of a malpractice suit presents you with an interesting situation. He will understandably have his guard up about this issue, particularly if you express dissatisfaction about your care. You want this interview to be as cordial and fair-minded as possible. You should find a way to assure your doctor that a lawsuit is the last thing on your mind; the first thing on your mind is your health. But, if you come into your doctor's office with well-marshaled arguments of why you should take a particular diagnostic test, he will realize that failing to give you this test may put him at some risk.

Finally, it may be helpful to bring a spouse, family member, or friend along to your appointment, since two voices and four ears are usually better than one voice and two ears. If you do bring someone else along, be sure to review your concerns and questions with that person before your appointment.

Getting Your Insurer to Pay for Your Test

Convincing your insurer to pay for an "unusual" test is not easy—luck helps. But your doctor can help too, especially if you have made a cogent case for why you are at special risk for a disease. If you have a good relationship with your doctor, she may go the extra mile to justify the test to your insurer.

Insurers themselves vary in their willingness to make exceptions to their rules about appropriate candidates for diagnostic tests. Here's where the luck comes in: These variations are not only from insurance company to insurance company, but from region to region. A large insurer may have very good customer relations in the New England area and poor customer relations in the Midwest.

If all else fails, and you have a complaint involving your claims, you can contact your state's Insurance Commissioner, who will review your claim. If the Insurance Commissioner finds that the insurance company has acted in an unlawful or unethical way, your insurer will have to compensate you.

Of course, one way to eliminate this hassle is to pay for the test yourself, out of your pocket. It may not seem reasonable, but in actuality, many of the tests we recommend here cost very little.

Maybe You've Got the Wrong Doctor

If your doctor does not make enough time for a discussion about diagnostic tests or if he refuses to give your arguments reasonable consideration, you should probably consider changing to another primary care doctor.

In an atmosphere dominated by managed care, we sometimes forget that we have this option. With the exception of people who live in very underserved areas, most of us have the ability to choose a primary care physician. In many cases, we also have the ability to choose specialists for problems out of the primary physician's area of expertise. When checking that your new physician participates in your health care plan, it's always a good idea to follow up with a call to the physician in question, since plan directories are not always up-to-date.

But is there any way to know ahead of time if a doctor will take your concerns seriously? First, ask around. The surest way to judge the quality of a physician is to ask his patients. Family members, friends, your health benefits officer at work, or the county or state medical society might suggest a particularly good physician in this regard. Better yet, if you know someone who works in a health care setting, you might be able to get an insider's perspective.

In addition to finding a physician who is open to unusual diagnostic testing, you'll want to decide what other physician characteristics are most important to you. It may be important to you to have a female or a male doctor, or one in a specific age range. Also, a physician's particular style of patient interaction may be

(continued on page 34)

THE LAST OBSTACLE TO TESTING

Along with your doctor and your insurer, there may be one more obstacle to getting diagnostic tests: *yourself*.

Embarrassment

Let's start with the relatively small stuff—embarrassment and discomfort. For example, the Pap test for cervical cancer involves a pelvic examination—hardly a picnic for the most secure woman. No fun. But the test can find signs of cervical cancer—a deadly disease—while the cancer is still treatable. It's a test that can save your life.

Sigmoidoscopic screening for colon cancer can be equally uncomfortable, requiring the placement of a small camera into the rectum and colon. Interestingly, one study found that patients waiting to have sigmoidoscopies anticipated embarrassment, discomfort, and pain. Afterward, however, they admitted that the test was not as bad as they had expected. So there's a good chance that your anticipation of a procedure is worse than the test itself.

Expense

We need to be honest here: Often (too often) you will end up having to foot the bill. But if your analysis has convinced you that you should have a particular test, you'll find that you *have* to find the money, even if it means restructuring your budget.

Inconvenience

Sometimes people don't get diagnostic tests because they do not want the aggravation of arguing with their doctor or pestering their insurer. There is no denying it; 9 times out of 10, this will entail some serious and endless phone calls, including lots of time on hold. Just remember, the trade-off is the possibility of catching a life-threatening disease. It's well worth it!

Too Much Worry

There are those of us who believe that there's really nothing that can be done to stop a disease once it has gotten hold of us. But in this book, we recommend tests that detect diseases that can be treated if diagnosed early.

Those of us who worry too much also tend to worry about worrying. For example, we know that getting a mammogram will ratchet up our general anxiety, so we avoid the whole business. That is perfectly understandable; it is also perfectly self-destructive. When the late singer Warren Zevon talked about his fatal lung cancer, he said sardonically, "I might have made a tactical error in not going to a physician for 20 years. It's one of those phobias that didn't pay off."

Too Little Worry

People who worry too little come from the tribe of dyed-in-the-wool deniers. These happy folk are of the school of thought that, "Yes, there are some awful diseases out there, but they won't get me!" Obviously, the younger and healthier you are, the less likely you are to take a screening test—no matter what your risk factors. But, of course, that is just whom these tests are for: people who do not exhibit symptoms!

Sobering Up the Psyche

The most important determinant of whether or not we opt for a test is whether or not our physician recommends it, plus our belief in the effectiveness of screening for the disease in question. This holds true when the doctor recommends the test and also if the doctor advises you not to receive a test. Still, in today's medical environment, your own evaluation should be the deciding factor. As we have seen, your doctor may not always know what is best for you when it comes to diagnostic tests.

crucial to you. You should also find out who else is in your prospective physician's group practice, since these are often the doctors who are on call if you need medical care when the clinic is not open.

Furthermore, determine which hospital your doctor admits patients to, and learn as much as you can about that hospital's track record. Practical concerns, like the location or operating hours of a physician's clinic, may also help you decide. While your required office visit copayment may be the same regardless of which physician in your health plan you use, rates may vary among doctors for ancillary services. Try to obtain information about your prospective doctor's billing practices.

You may also want to determine how long this physician has been in practice, with the understanding that this is not always a reliable indicator of physician quality. Generally speaking, the longer a physician has been in practice, the more likely she has obtained experience treating medical problems similar to your own. Of course, the more recently a physician has graduated from medical school, the more current her medical knowledge may be. Medicine is a very rapidly evolving profession that demands that its practitioners stay up-to-date. If your treatment requires surgery, you will want to ask your prospective physician about her experience regarding that procedure.

You can do additional research in the Directory of Medical Specialists, which has biographical information, such as medical school and residency program attended, of approximately 400,000 doctors. Alternatively, the American Medical Association (AMA) has a free online service called AMA Physician Select, which provides information about physicians in your geographical area (www.ama-assn.org/aps/amahg.htm). It may also be useful to contact your state's Medical Licensing Board or Department of Insurance in order to inquire whether any sanctions or disciplinary actions have been taken against the physician in question.

A visit to a physician's clinic can be quite revealing. Take note of the office atmosphere. Is this clinic organized and clean? Are the support staff members friendly and helpful, and do they respond appropriately to problems with patients? The level of professionalism exhibited by the office staff is often a reflection of the level of professionalism of the physicians running that office.

Many physicians will offer free consultation visits for prospective patients during which much of the above information can be obtained. This is the ideal time for you to express your interest and concern with diagnostic tests. Level with him and get him to level with you. Is he flexible on this issue? If not, keep looking.

TWO

THE CONDITIONS

ABDOMINAL AORTIC ANEURYSM

An abdominal aortic aneurysm (AAA) is a bulge in the descending aorta, the main blood vessel coming from the heart that supplies blood to all of the organs in your abdomen and to your legs. The normal diameter of the aorta is about 1 inch (2.4 centimeters) or less. An AAA is defined as a dilation (swelling) of the aorta greater than 3 centimeters. An aneurysm on the abdominal aorta may continue to grow larger until it bursts and causes massive internal bleeding.

More than 90 percent of AAAs are associated with atherosclerosis and can cause leg pain, numbness, or fatigue. Unfortunately, most people who have an AAA do not experience any symptoms until it expands or bursts, resulting in bleeding and often, rapid death. The larger an aneurysm becomes, the easier it is for it to grow bigger still. Abdominal aortic aneurysm is not a condition you hear about every day. Yet two Mayo Clinic studies show a threefold increase in this disorder over the past 40 years. The increase may be partly due to the upsurge in smoking since World War II. Also, as more people live longer, this type of aneurysm occurs more frequently. Abdominal aortic aneurysms occur in 5 to 7 percent of people over the age of 60 in the United States, mostly males. About 15,000 Americans die each year from ruptured AAAs.

Compared with the half million who die annually of heart attacks, the number of deaths due to aneurysms is small. However, because rupture causes such a massive loss of blood, the mortality rate from AAA rupture is very high. About 62 percent of people who experience a ruptured AAA die before they reach the hospital. Of those who do reach the hospital and have emergency surgery, only about 50 percent survive. Therefore, a ruptured AAA means death over 80 percent of the time. If detected early, however, surgery eliminates this silent danger 95 percent of the time.

Risk Factors

MODIFIABLE

Cigarette smoking: A number of studies have shown that cigarette smoking is an important risk factor for AAA (probably because it causes atherosclerosis).

High blood pressure: Untreated high blood pressure increases your risk for AAA.

NONMODIFIABLE

Age: AAA is found most often after 55 to 60 years of age. In fact, it has been estimated to occur in 52 of every 100,000 men between the ages of 55 and 64, but this rate shoots up to 409 of every 100,000 men over age 80. Obviously, the total number of patients with AAA will increase as the population ages.

Atherosclerosis: The most common underlying cause of an AAA is atherosclerosis. This is the gradual process in which cholesterol and scar tissue build up, forming plaque on the walls of our arteries. Since plaque formation can weaken and damage the walls of the arteries, it makes them more vulnerable to an aneurysm. Anyone with a diagnosis of atherosclerosis is at heightened risk for an AAA.

Ehlers-Danlos Syndromes: This is a group of relatively rare syndromes that share common features, including connective tissue disorders. People with these syndromes have an increased risk of an AAA.

Family history of AAA: If you have one or more first-degree relatives with an AAA, your likelihood of incurring this disease rises to 12–19 percent.

Gender: AAAs are four times more common in men than women.

Your Risk Level

The three most significant risk factors for AAA are age (over 60), gender (male), and a family history of the disease. As always, any combination of these (and the other risk factors listed above) multiplies your composite risk, and should be considered in your decision as to whether or not you should be tested for the presence of an AAA.

Tests You May Want to Request

When a physician uses **abdominal palpation,** he'll feel your abdomen for irregularities. The statistical accuracy of physical examination in detecting AAA is not completely known. Large aneurysms are easier to detect than small ones, and it is easier to detect aneurysms in thin people.

Auscultation—listening to an AAA with a stethoscope—reveals sounds like a blowing or a whooshing (called a bruit).

These tests are not necessarily reliable, and with a condition as dangerous as an AAA, it could be extremely risky to depend on these physical examinations.

If you have any of the significant risk factors for AAA, you may want to consider having an **abdominal ultrasound**—an inexpensive, noninvasive, and accurate test. See page 143 for more information.

BLADDER CANCER

Your bladder is located in your lower abdomen and receives and stores urine coming from your kidneys until you eventually excrete it. In adulthood, new bladder cells are constantly produced to replace those that die of old age or disease. Normally, division of cells is under very tight control and is mediated by the genes inside each cell. If the genes are damaged, the control over cell division may be lost in one particular cell, and a cancer cell is formed.

Bladder cancer occurs in many different forms, but it usually originates in the bladder lining. The tumor is categorized as either low stage (superficial) or high stage (muscle invasive) at diagnosis.

Each year in the United States, there are 52,000 new cases of bladder cancer, and it causes approximately 13,000 deaths. It accounts for about 7 percent of all new cancers.

Risk Factors

MODIFIABLE

Cigarette smoking: Cigarette smoking increases the risk of bladder cancer three times over that of nonsmokers. It is estimated that about 50 percent of these cancers in men and 30 percent in women are due to smoking. If you quit smoking, the risk decreases after 5 years and nears normal at 15 years.

NONMODIFIABLE

Age: Ninety-nine percent of people who get bladder cancer are over age 40, with the average age being 68. Rates in those age 70 years and older are approximately two to three times higher than those in people ages 55 to 69 years, and about 15 to 20 times higher than rates for people ages 30 to 54. In men 75 years of age or older, bladder cancer is the fifth leading cause of cancer death.

Bladder polyps: A history of bladder polyps increases risk of bladder cancer.

Chronic bladder inflammation: A history of recurrent urinary tract infections and urinary stones increases risk of bladder cancer.

Ethnicity: Bladder cancer is more common in Caucasians than in Hispanics or African-Americans. The rates for black men and Hispanic men are similar and are about one-half the white, non-Hispanic rate. Lowest rates for bladder cancer are found in the Asian populations. For women, the highest rates are also in white non-Hispanics and are about twice the rate for Hispanics. Black women, however, have higher rates than Hispanic women.

Family history: Having one first-degree relative (parent or sibling) with bladder cancer almost doubles your risk.

Gender: Bladder cancer is three times more common in men than women.

Medications history: Past use of medications like phenacetin (not available in the United States) and chemotherapy agents like cyclophosphamide and chlornaphazin can increase the risk of bladder cancer.

Past carcinogen exposure: Occupational exposures may account for up to 25 percent of all bladder cancers. Most of the risk is due to exposure to a group of chemicals known as arylamines. Occupations with high exposure to arylamines include dye workers, rubber workers, leather workers, truck drivers, painters, and aluminum workers. Because of their association with bladder cancer, some arylamines have been eliminated or greatly reduced in occupational settings. It often takes as long as 20 years after exposure (called a latent period) for bladder cancer to develop.

Your Risk Level

Risk Factor	Number of Points
Age 50 to 59	1
Age 60 to 69	2
Age 70 or older	3
Have one first-degree relative with bladder cancer	3
Have two first-degree relatives with bladder cancer	3
Have had past exposure to arylamine	4
Smoker: 20 pack-years or more	4
History of bladder polyps	4
History of chronic bladder inflammation	3
Past use of a phenacetin	2
Past treatment with cyclophosphamide or chlornaphazin	2

Total Points	Lifetime Risk of Bladder Cancer
0–4	Low
5–8	Moderate
9 or more	High

Tests You May Want to Consider

Evaluation of the bladder for the presence of bladder cancer is performed most often by a urologist.

Cystoscopy enables the urologist to directly view the inside of the urinary bladder in great detail using a cystoscope. This test is invasive and expensive, and is therefore not cost-effective as a screening test in patients with no symptoms.

Urine cytology is an examination of the urine to screen for cancer cells. This test has a very low sensitivity for diagnosing bladder cancer (typically about 30 percent). Upper tract evaluations, too, are not reliable for screening for bladder cancer.

We recommend the **NMP22 test**—a very new test for bladder cancer. Turn to page 207 for more information.

BREAST CANCER

Except for nonmelanoma skin cancers, breast cancer is the most common cancer among women. It is estimated that this year about 211,300 new cases of invasive breast cancer will be diagnosed among women in the United States, and 1,300 cases will be diagnosed in men. About 39,800 women are expected to die from it. About 55,700 cases of noninvasive breast cancer (DCIS) are diagnosed in United States women each year.

Breast cancer is the second leading cause of cancer death in women, exceeded only by lung cancer. It is believed that earlier detection and treatment have led to the recent decline in death rates from breast cancer.

Though far less common than for women, it is possible for men to develop breast cancer. In the year 2000, the American Cancer Society estimated that 1,400 new cases of invasive breast cancer were diagnosed in men and approximately 400 men died from it, accounting for between 1 and 2 percent of all breast cancers.

There are several different types of breast cancer, some more dangerous than others. Nearly all breast cancers start in glandular tissue, such as in the lobules (milk-producing glands) or ducts (milk passages) of the breast. These two main types of breast cancer are referred to as ductal carcinomas and lobular carcinomas.

In ductal carcinomas, the cancer starts from one of the cells lining the ducts of the breast. The most common type of ductal carcinoma is referred to as ductal carcinoma *in situ* (DCIS). In DCIS, the cancer has not invaded the surrounding tissue of the breast, and nearly all women diagnosed at this early stage of breast cancer can be cured.

In contrast, infiltrating (or invasive) ductal carcinoma (IDC) is a cancer that starts from one of the cells lining the ducts of the breast, but has broken through the wall of the duct and invaded the surrounding fatty tissue of the breast. At this point, it can metastasize, or spread to other parts of the body. About 80 percent of invasive breast cancers are IDCs.

Risk Factors

MODIFIABLE

Cigarette smoking: Smoking increases a woman's chance of developing breast cancer.

Hormone replacement therapy (HRT): After menopause, women begin to have an increased risk of developing osteoporosis, heart disease, and possibly colorectal cancer. This is thought to be related to the postmenopausal decline in ovarian estrogen, and many postmenopausal women take estrogen supplements to prevent the development of these diseases.

However, HRT studies also show that there are risks in taking these supplements. For example, many studies have suggested that women taking HRT had a small, but real, increase in the lifetime risk of breast cancer, as well as an increased risk of uterine cancer and stroke. This increase in risk seemed particularly true if the women were on estrogen supplementation for more than 10 years.

Follow-up studies suggested that adding progestin (a drug that mimics progesterone) to the estrogen supplements removed the increased risk of uterine cancer, but this did not decrease the risk of breast cancer and stroke.

Recently, the issue has become far more complex and controversial, as findings have cast the cardiovascular benefits of HRT into serious doubt. The results of the Heart and Estrogen/Progestin Replacement Study follow-up (HERS II), released in 2002, found that there were *no overall* cardiovascular benefits over a 7-year period in postmenopausal women already diagnosed with coronary heart disease using an estrogen/progestin combination. Furthermore, the results of the Women's Health Initiative, released in 2002, showed that postmenopausal women without CHD who took estrogen/progestin pills for over 5 years also received no cardiovascular benefit. The evidence is still good, however, that postmenopausal estrogen supplementation can help prevent osteoporosis.

Postmenopausal women who are considering estrogen supplementation for cardiovascular benefits should talk with their gynecologists on the most recent findings regarding HRT therapies in postmenopausal women.

Weight: The link between weight and breast cancer risk is controversial. Several new studies suggest that overweight (obese) women who gained weight as adults are at an increased risk of developing breast cancer, but women who have been overweight since childhood are not at any significantly higher risk.

NONMODIFIABLE

Age: A woman's risk of breast cancer increases with age, as shown in the table below. About 77 percent of women with breast cancer are over age 50 at the time of diagnosis, but only 0.3 percent of all breast cancer cases in the United States occur in women between the ages of 20 and 29.

Female Age and Breast Cancer Incidence

By age 30	1 out of 2,212
By age 40	1 out of 235
By age 50	1 out of 54
By age 60	1 out of 23
By age 70	1 out of 14
By age 80	1 out of 10
Ever	1 out of 8

Breast Cancer Gene 1 (BRCA1) and Breast Cancer Gene 2 (BRCA2) mutations: The normal role of BRCA genes 1 and 2 in our body is to repair damaged DNA in our cells; therefore, mutation of these genes (which impairs their ability to fix DNA) can allow cancer to develop. In 1994, researchers discovered that women who carry mutations of BRCA1 or BRCA2 are at higher risk of developing breast cancer than women who do not have these genetic mutations.

But how much higher is the risk? Many specialists in the genetics of breast cancer have suggested that women with BRCA gene mutations have a lifetime probability of getting breast cancer that exceeds 80 percent. Other studies dispute this estimate, arguing that the risk is not that high.

For example, in a study published in August 2002 in the *Journal of the National Cancer Institute*, Colin Begg, Ph.D., of Memorial Sloan-Kettering Cancer Center in New York said this 80 percent risk rate cannot be applied to every woman with mutations of the BRCA genes. "It is likely that the typical mutation carrier would have risks lower than that," said Dr. Begg. He continued, "The risks that have been quoted are among the highest, because they have been based on studies using high-risk families."

Although the exact increase in breast cancer risk associated with BRCA mutations cannot be stated with certainty, we do know that women with BRCA gene mutations have a risk higher than the lifetime risk of 11 to 12 percent for the general female population in the United States. Yet it clearly varies with ethnic groups: A study of mutation carriers in Iceland found a 20 percent risk, while a similar study among Ashkenazi Jews found a 56 percent lifetime risk.

If a daughter has a parent with a known BRCA1 or BRCA2 mutation, she has a 50 percent chance of inheriting the altered

BRCA AND OVARIAN CANCER

Breast cancer is not the only cancer that can arise in women with a BRCA gene mutation. Women with BRCA1 and -2 gene mutations are also thought to have a 15 to 65 percent risk of developing ovarian cancer by age 70, compared to a 1 to 2 percent overall lifetime risk in women without these mutations.

In the May 3, 2000 issue of the *Journal of the American Medical Association*, researchers reported on the increased risks of ovarian cancer in women carrying BRCA1 and -2 gene mutations. This particular study was restricted to Ashkenazi Jewish women. Of the 189 patients treated for ovarian cancer during a 12-month period, 88 were found have a BRCA1 or BRCA2 gene mutation.

The researchers also found that women with BRCA mutations did not typically develop ovarian cancer until they were almost 60 years of age or older, and very few women with BRCA gene mutations developed ovarian cancer until after age 40. These findings provide hope for young women who want to keep their ovaries intact early in life so they can have children. After having their children, they can then consider the possibility of having their ovaries removed to greatly reduce their chances of getting ovarian cancer.

BRCA IN MEN

If you are a male who actually has been diagnosed with breast cancer, you should consider BRCA testing for two reasons: to assess your risk of recurrent breast cancer, and to assess the breast cancer risk of your sisters and daughters.

BRCA gene and an increased likelihood to develop cancer. Similarly, if through genetic testing she finds she has inherited the mutation, she has a 50 percent chance of passing it on to her children.

Childbirth status: Women who had their first child after age 30 or who have never had a full-term pregnancy are at a higher risk for developing breast cancer. The protective effect of having children early in life is due to both the absence of menstrual cycles during pregnancy and lactation and some permanent decrease in estrogen responsiveness in breast cells.

Ethnicity: Certain Jewish populations are at particularly high risk for mutations in the BRCA genes, and thus breast and ovarian cancer. Recent studies have shown that there are three specific mutations of the BRCA1 and BRCA2 genes (called founder mutations) that are more common in Jews of Eastern European origin (Ashkenazi Jews). About 1 out of 40 Ashkenazi Jews carry a founder mutation, as do about 20 percent of Jewish women diagnosed with breast cancer before age 41. Most significantly, Ashkenazi Jews carrying a mutation have a 56 percent lifetime risk of breast cancer.

Exposure to mutagenic substances in the environment: Most DNA mutations that result in breast cancer are probably caused by exposure to various mutagenic substances in the environment. These substances include chemicals found in the environment that mimic the effects of estrogen (environmental estrogens), high dose radiation, carcinogens (cancer-causing substances) consumed in the diet, and overexposure to the carcinogens in cigarette smoke. Without doubt, there are many others that remain unknown. It is believed that about 90 percent of all breast cancers are the result of sporadic mutations in our DNA.

Family history of breast cancer but no BRCA gene mutations: Only about 10 percent of all breast cancers are thought to be due to a genetic predisposition to breast cancer—the other 90 percent of cases are simply sporadic. Of the 10 percent that are due to genetic predisposition, only about half of them are due to mutations in BRCA1 or -2 genes.

Therefore, about half the families that show a genetic predisposition to breast cancer do not carry either BRCA gene mutation. They almost certainly have some genetic anomaly, but scientists have yet to discover it. If you have a strong family history of breast cancer (onset prior to age 45, two or more first-degree relatives affected) and you test negative for BRCA gene mutations, you should still increase monitoring for early signs of breast cancer.

Gender: Breast cancer is almost exclusively a women's disease. However, in the year 2000, the American Cancer Society estimated that 1,400 new cases of invasive breast cancer were diagnosed in men and approximately 400 men died from it. We mention it here because if a male breast cancer is in your immediate family, it is particularly suggestive of the presence of a BRCA2 gene mutation.

Menstrual cycles: Women who begin menstruating at an early age (before age 12) and those who reach menopause after age 50 have an increased risk of breast cancer. Each menstrual cycle is associated with significant elevations in levels of estrogen, and exposure to estrogen increases the risk of breast cancer. Thus, the greater the total number of menstrual cycles in a woman's life, the greater her total estrogen exposure and her risk of developing breast cancer.

Personal history: Women who have had breast cancer in one breast are three to four times as likely to develop breast cancer in the other breast than women who have never had breast cancer.

Your Risk Level

We have developed the following table to help women estimate their lifetime risk of acquiring breast cancer, based on known risk factors.

Risk Factor	Number of Points
Used HRT for more than 10 years	2
Have been obese since childhood	2
Smoker: more than 20 pack-years	2
Between ages 51 and 60	2
Older than age 60	3
Began menstruating at a young age or entered menopause at a late age	2
Delayed pregnancy	2
Of Eastern European Jewish ancestry (Ashkenazi)	4
Have one first-degree relative with breast cancer	3
Have two or more first-degree relatives with breast cancer	7
Have a male in the family with breast cancer	5
Known carrier of BRCA gene mutation(s)	9

Total Points	Lifetime Risk of Breast Cancer
0–4	Low
5–8	Moderate
9 or more	High

The most frequently used option for those who are at high risk for breast cancer is to become extremely vigilant about detecting the early development of breast cancer. In particular, this means frequent **screening mammograms**.

In 1996, the American Society of Clinical Oncology recommended that only women with a strong family history of breast cancer or those who have developed breast cancer at an early age may be eligible for **BRCA genetic testing**. Since BRCA gene mutations also increase ovarian cancer risk, a strong family history of this cancer can also justify BRCA gene testing. Candidates for BRCA testing generally include the following:

- Breast cancer in two or more close relatives, such as a mother and two sisters
- Early onset of breast cancer in family members, often before age 50
- History of breast cancer in more than one generation
- Cancer in both breasts in one or more family members
- Frequent occurrence of ovarian cancer
- One or more BRCA-positive relatives
- Eastern and Central European (Ashkenazi) Jewish ancestry, with a family history of breast or ovarian cancer

If you feel that you would be a good candidate for BRCA testing, see page 155 for more information.

CAROTID ARTERY DISEASE
AND STROKE

Carotid artery disease (CAD) is a disorder that affects the large blood vessels leading to the head and brain (carotid arteries). Like those of the heart, the brain's cells need a constant supply of oxygen-rich blood. This blood supply is delivered to the brain by the two carotid arteries in the front of your neck and by two smaller arteries at the back of your neck. All of these arteries can develop atherosclerosis—a buildup of plaque. If blood flow to the brain is obstructed to any degree, the brain begins to lose its energy supply, and brain cells become injured. And if blood is obstructed for more than several minutes, the brain cell injury can be permanent. The loss or alteration of bodily function that results is called a stroke.

Ischemic stroke is the most common type of stroke and usually occurs when an artery to the brain becomes blocked for some reason. Less often, it can be caused by an episode of severely low blood pressure (hypotensive stroke) or low blood oxygen (hypoxic stroke).

The signs and symptoms of a stroke must last for at least 24 hours for the episode to be considered a stroke. On occasion, an individual with temporarily reduced blood flow to the brain will develop related symptoms that last less than 24 hours—a condition called a transient ischemic attack (TIA) or ministroke. The specific symptoms of a TIA or stroke depend upon which portion of the brain has been damaged.

In one of the most common stroke scenarios, a piece of plaque breaks off from the carotid artery, travels to an artery that supplies blood to a major portion of the brain, and plugs the artery. Blockage of this artery can damage portions of the brain that control voluntary muscles and sensation in the face, arms, hands, and sometimes legs. Hence, along with the typical dizziness or loss of consciousness, damage to this area of the brain can result in temporary or permanent paralysis and loss of sensation in these areas. Blockage of this artery can also destroy important language-processing centers, making it difficult for the patient to produce or understand speech.

By far, the most common cause of ischemic stroke is carotid artery disease (CAD). In fact, it has been estimated that up to 50 percent of all ischemic strokes are due to the presence of CAD. In this disorder, the carotid arteries become too narrow due to plaque formation. Blockage can occur if plaque breaks off and plugs an artery in the brain, or if blood flowing over the plaque produces a blood clot which then travels to the brain and blocks an artery. In addition, ischemic stroke can be caused by blood clots forming in the heart and then traveling to the brain. Increased risk for this latter type of ischemic stroke sometimes occurs as a result of an irregular heartbeat, a heart attack, or abnormalities of the heart valves.

It's important to remember that stroke is the third leading cause of death in the United States and a principal cause of long-term disability in much of the industrialized world. In the United States, about 600,000 people suffer from a new or recurrent stroke annually, and stroke is a contributing factor in 150,000 deaths each year.

If you find you have CAD, not only are you at much greater

risk for an ischemic stroke, but you may have coronary heart disease as well. The atherosclerotic process that builds up plaque in the carotid arteries is very similar to the process in the coronary arteries.

Risk Factors

MODIFIABLE

Cigarette smoking: Many studies have shown smoking to be an important risk factor for stroke. The carbon monoxide and other chemicals in cigarette smoke damage the cardiovascular system in many ways. The use of oral contraceptives combined with cigarette smoking increases stroke risk even further.

Drug abuse: People who abuse intravenous drugs carry a high risk of stroke. Also, cocaine use has been closely related to strokes, heart attacks, and a variety of other cardiovascular complications.

Dyslipidemia: People with high triglyceride levels, low HDL ("good") and high LDL ("bad") cholesterol levels have an increased risk of ischemic stroke.

Excessive alcohol intake: Although moderate alcohol intake appears to decrease the risk of heart disease and stroke, excessive drinking (average of more than one drink per day for women and more than two drinks per day for men) and binge drinking can raise blood pressure, cholesterol, contribute to obesity, and increase risk of stroke.

High blood pressure: High blood pressure is probably the most important modifiable risk factor for stroke. In fact, stroke risk increases directly with the degree of elevation of blood pressure. It is believed that the effective treatment of high blood pressure in the past decade is a key reason for the recent decline in stroke rates.

Obesity: The incidence of stroke is greater in people who are overweight.

Nonmodifiable

Age: Ischemic stroke is certainly more common as you get older, but it is important to recognize that one-third of all strokes occur in people under 65 years of age. The overall incidence increases sharply with age in both sexes. In people over the age of 55, the incidence of stroke doubles for each decade of life up to the age of 90, when the pattern reverses itself—in other words, if you make it past 90 and haven't had a stroke, you probably never will.

Carotid artery disease: The presence of significant carotid artery disease puts you at higher risk for having an ischemic stroke. Also, be aware that if you find you have significant blockage in your carotid arteries, you should have your coronary arteries evaluated as well.

Diabetes: Diabetes is an independent risk factor for stroke. This may be because diabetics have significantly higher rates of atherosclerosis and high blood pressure, which are important risk factors. People with diabetes also often have high cholesterol and are overweight, increasing their risk even more.

Ethnicity: African-Americans have a much higher risk of disability and death from a stroke, in part because they have a greater incidence of high blood pressure, a major stroke risk factor.

Family history of stroke: The chance of stroke is greater in people who have a family history of stroke.

Gender: The overall incidence of stroke is 30 percent higher in men than in women. However, the incidence is very similar after advanced age (70 to 80).

History of transient ischemic attacks (TIAs): TIAs are mini-strokes with temporary stroke symptoms, like tingling in the face and limbs, or an inability to speak. They are strong predictors of stroke. A person who has had one or more TIAs is almost 10 times more likely to have a stroke than someone of the same age and sex who has not.

Irregular heartbeats, particularly atrial fibrillation: Although these individuals are at greater than average risk for ischemic stroke, duplex ultrasound (the test we recommend) will *not* identify this risk since clot formation originates in the heart and not the carotid arteries. An electrocardiogram (ECG) is needed to find electrical problems in the heart.

Personal history of stroke: Approximately one-third of all stroke survivors will have another stroke within 5 years.

Your Risk Level

When assessing the risk of stroke, it is important to remember that the greater the number and severity of known risk factors you have, the greater your overall risk of stroke. Calculating personal risk for stroke, or any other medical disorder, is an inexact science. All we can really do is gather information about our known risks and make an educated guess. If, for example, you have a long history of hypertension and have previously exhibited transient ischemic attack (TIA; ministroke) symptoms, and you have other risk factors as well, it would certainly make good sense to be tested further. If you are a slightly overweight male over 55 with one grandfather who suffered from a stroke, you may or may not think this combination of risk factors warrants concern—that is, enough concern to seriously consider having a diagnostic test for the presence of carotid artery disease.

Only you can decide whether to have this test, based on your risk factors for stroke. However, keep in mind that if you have a stroke and survive it, you may lose your ability to walk, speak, and live a normal life. In fact, around 25 percent of those people who survive a stroke end up in a nursing home for the remainder of their lives.

Stroke risk factors should not be taken lightly. Get tested if you are at risk, and know the symptoms of a mild stroke (because if

you have one, you are at much greater risk for having a more severe one later).

- Sudden numbness or weakness of face, arm, or leg, especially
  on one side of the body
- Sudden confusion or trouble speaking or understanding speech
- Sudden trouble seeing in one or both eyes
- Sudden trouble walking, dizziness, or loss of balance or coordi-
  nation
- Sudden severe headache with no known cause

Tests You May Want to Consider

There are a number of tests that are commonly used to detect
carotid artery disease, and they vary widely in reliability, cost, and
invasiveness.

Cerebral angiography is considered to be the gold standard for
detecting carotid artery disease, but it is very invasive and expensive. It's best used to confirm a diagnosis of CAD, rather than as
an initial screening test. Cerebral angiography does carry significant health risks, including stroke, allergic reaction to the contrast
dye used, and kidney failure. It is because of these risks and high
costs that cerebral angiography is increasingly being replaced by
other tests.

MRA (Magnetic Resonance Angiography) is an excellent
imaging procedure for the carotid arteries, but it is relatively expensive. It is more time-consuming and less widely available than
other tests. Furthermore, the MRA cannot be performed in patients
who are critically ill, unable to lie down flat, have claustrophobia,
or have cardiac pacemakers or other implanted ferromagnetic devices. In fact, as many as 17 percent of MRA studies cannot be successfully completed because the patient is unable to lie flat and still
for the duration of the test.

In some cases, doctors can tell if you have carotid artery disease during a normal checkup. By **auscultation**—placing a stethoscope over the carotid artery in your neck—your doctor can listen for a rushing sound, called a bruit. The results of this test can be misleading, however. Bruit sounds may not always be present, even when carotid artery disease is severe. Also, your doctor cannot determine the extent of blockage through this test. So even if auscultation suggests that you have carotid artery disease, further testing is always in order.

Computed tomography angiography (CTA) uses CT scanning (x-rays) to visualize blood flow in arterial vessels. Although CTA can also provide excellent pictures of the carotid arteries on its own, it usually involves injection of a contrast dye into a vein to better visualize the blood vessels. Some patients can suffer from allergic reactions or acute kidney failure due to reactions to the dye. This procedure is also quite expensive, and involves exposure to x-ray radiation, so we don't recommend it as a first screening test for carotid artery disease.

We believe that of all the tests available, the **duplex ultrasound** is the best screening tool for carotid artery disease in asymptomatic people. It is a very safe test, is accurate, and involves no radiation exposure or dye injection. It's also relatively inexpensive. See page 174 for more information.

In addition, you should also consider the tests we suggest for coronary heart disease (blood glucose tests for type 2 diabetes, the blood tests for hemochromatosis, the EBCT scan, the ITST, plasma homocysteine, and the C-reactive protein test). All of these tests check for the presence of atherosclerosis—a cause of coronary heart disease and CAD.

COLORECTAL CANCER

If cancer begins in the colon, it is called colon cancer, and if it begins in the rectum, it is called rectal cancer. Either of these conditions may also be called colorectal cancer. The vast majority of colorectal cancers arise from polyps, growths that can form on the lining of the large intestine. Most of the time these polyps are benign (harmless), but when they are the type known as adenomatous polyps, they can turn into cancer. This is a slow process, taking between 5 and 15 years, which allows for plenty of time to intervene before a true colorectal cancer develops.

Colorectal cancer is the second leading cause of cancer-related deaths in the United States. Only lung cancer claims more lives. Each year, approximately 150,000 Americans are diagnosed with colorectal cancer and 50,000 die. Eighty to 90 million Americans (approximately 25 percent of the United States population) are considered at risk because of age or other factors.

Risk Factors

MODIFIABLE

Cigarette smoking: Smoking has long been associated with many kinds of cancer. The American Cancer Society (ACS) and the

National Cancer Institute (NCI) have recently added colorectal cancer to the list. An ACS study showed that smoking for 20 years or more increases the risk of dying from cancer of the colon or rectum by more than 40 percent.

Diet and lifestyle: Colorectal cancer seems to be associated with diets that are high in red meat and total calories. People who have a sedentary lifestyle or are obese have an increased risk of developing the disease.

Alcohol consumption: Some studies have shown that heavy alcohol consumption increases the risk of colorectal cancer.

NONMODIFIABLE

Age: Ninety percent of people diagnosed with colorectal cancer are over 50 years old. However, it's important to understand that people in their 30s and 40s may begin growing the precancerous polyps that will eventually become colorectal cancer.

Ethnicity: Colorectal cancer rates show wide divergence by ethnic group, with rates in the Alaska Native population over four times as high as rates in the American Indian population for both men and women.

After Alaska Natives, the next highest rates are among people of Japanese descent, followed by African-Americans and non-Hispanic Caucasians.

Familial adenomatous polyposis: A rare, inherited condition, familial adenomatous polyposis (FAP) causes hundreds of polyps to form in the colon and rectum. Unless this condition is treated, it is almost certain to lead to colorectal cancer.

Family history: Anyone with a first-degree relative (parents, siblings, children) who has had colorectal cancer is more likely to develop this type of cancer, especially if the relative had the cancer at a young age (45 years old or younger). If more than one family member has had colorectal cancer, the chances increase even more. People with a strong family history of colorectal cancer not only should get a screening colonoscopy, but also should consider genetic testing for a disorder called hereditary nonpolyposis colorectal cancer (HNPCC), which accounts for about 3 to 5 percent of all colorectal cancers. People who carry the abnormal gene for HNPCC have up to an 80 percent lifetime risk of developing colorectal cancer (see Hereditary Nonpolyposis Colorectal Cancer, on page 90).

Gender: Even though research has suggested that women may develop colorectal cancer at an older age than men, the American College of Gastroenterology has concluded that women should *not* delay screening.

History of inflammatory bowel disease: Anyone with a history of inflammatory bowel disease, such as ulcerative colitis or Crohn's disease, is at increased risk for colorectal cancer.

AN OUNCE OF PREVENTION

As with all serious diseases, the most favorable outcome is to never get the disease at all. In this regard, studies of average-risk people suggest that regular use of acetaminophen, nonsteroidal anti-inflammatory drugs (NSAIDs) like ibuprofen, folic acid, calcium supplements, and estrogen for postmenopausal women may inhibit the development of colorectal cancer. (If you take calcium supplements, be sure to buy brands that include vitamin D to facilitate effective absorption of calcium from the intestine.)

Taking a single baby aspirin each day may also be effective in preventing colorectal cancer, as it appears to prevent the growth of the type of polyp that develops into colorectal cancer. In fact, in one study, a single daily baby aspirin reduced the risk that precancerous polyps would recur in patients by almost 20 percent.

History of intestinal polyps: Polyps, growths on the inner wall of the colon and rectum, are fairly common in people over age 50. If a polyp is an adenomatous polyp, there is a strong likelihood of it becoming cancerous. But even if only benign polyps are found in a routine colonoscopy, patients should return for repeat colonoscopies every 3 years.

History of previous cancers: Research shows that women with a history of cancer of the ovary, uterus, or breast have a somewhat increased chance of developing colorectal cancer. Also, a person who has already had colorectal cancer is at increased risk for developing this disease a second time.

Persistent undiagnosed symptoms: Any of the following symptoms, if not diagnosed as resulting from some other condition, may be a symptom of colorectal cancer: fatigue; persistent diarrhea; persistent constipation, rectal bleeding, change in frequency or appearance of bowel movements, weight loss, anemia, and abdominal pain.

Your Risk Level

Following the general rule, the more risk factors you have for colorectal cancer, the greater your risk. However, it is important to note that nearly 75 percent of all cases of colorectal cancer are diagnosed in people with no known risk factors other than their age. Therefore, being over age 50 alone is a significant enough risk to warrant testing.

Risk Factor	Number of Points
Older than 50 years of age	3
One first-degree relative diagnosed with colorectal cancer	3
Two affected first-degree relatives	5
One first-degree relative affected under age 45	5

(continued on page 66)

Risk Factor	Number of Points
Two first-degree relatives affected under age 45	9
Smoker: 20 pack-years or more	1
History of inflammatory bowel disease	3
History of intestinal polyps	3
Diet high in red meat	1
History of heavy alcohol intake	1

Total Points	Lifetime Risk of Colorectal Cancer
0–4	Low
5–8	Moderate
9 or more	High

Tests You May Want to Consider

In order to detect colon cancer or polyps in the colon, a number of tests are typically offered. A **digital rectal exam** only checks the first few inches of your rectum for polyps or tumors. Although safe and painless, it cannot detect problems with your upper rectum and colon.

The **fecal occult blood test** simply identifies blood in your stool. It is unreliable for detecting colorectal cancer, however, as blood in the stool can be a sign of any of a number of digestive tract problems. Not all cancers cause bleeding; precancerous polyps even more rarely cause bleeding and so are almost never found with this test.

A **barium enema** allows your doctor to evaluate your entire large intestine with an x-ray. Barium, a contrast dye, is placed into your bowel in an enema form. The barium fills and coats the lining of the bowel, creating a clear silhouette of your rectum, colon, and sometimes a small portion of your small intestine. This test is not only extremely uncomfortable, but can easily miss smaller polyps and "flat" cancers.

Sigmoidoscopy involves passing an endoscope through the rectum and up the colon as far as the sigmoid colon, allowing it to examine approximately the last 2 feet of your colon. Unfortunately, nearly half of all colorectal cancers occur beyond the sigmoid colon, and they cannot be found with this test.

A **colonoscopy**—the test we recommend for early detection of colorectal cancer—is similar to a sigmoidoscopy, but the endoscope is longer and is passed up the entire length of the colon, so the procedure can find early signs of cancer in the entire colon. It also enables the physician to see inflamed tissue, other abnormal growths, ulcers, and bleeding. For more information on this procedure, see page 169.

CORONARY HEART DISEASE

Cardiovascular disease (CVD) refers to any disorder that affects the heart muscle or the blood vessels of the heart. It includes conditions like coronary heart disease (CHD), congestive heart failure, congenital heart disease, and problems with the "electrical" properties of the heart. Coronary heart disease (also known as coronary artery disease) is the most prevalent form of CVD.

In CHD, the coronary arteries of the heart (which supply the heart muscle with blood) become narrowed or blocked by a gradual buildup of plaque within the artery wall, which reduces blood flow to the heart muscle. This process of building up plaque in arteries is termed atherosclerosis. It is a very complex process that involves many factors in the arteries, including inflammation and the accumulation of fats, like cholesterol. When it occurs in the coronary arteries and causes CHD, it can produce heart attacks.

To give you an idea of just how pervasive CHD is today, consider these recent statistics.

• CHD remains the single largest killer of both males and females in the United States.

• About 250,000 people a year suffer a fatal heart attack in the

United States. For nearly 50 percent of these people, it was their first and last symptom of CHD.

Risk Factors for CHD

MODIFIABLE

Cholesterol and triglycerides: The following blood levels are associated with increased risk of developing CHD.

- Total cholesterol over 240 mg/dl
- LDL (bad) cholesterol over 150 mg/dl
- Triglycerides over 150 mg/dl
- HDL (good) cholesterol *under* 40 mg/dl

Cigarette smoking: Smoking greatly increases your risk of getting CHD. In addition, people who smoke have more than twice the risk of having a heart attack compared with nonsmokers. Furthermore, that heart attack is two to four times more likely to be fatal (death in less than 2 hours) in smokers, compared to nonsmokers. Stopping smoking reduces this risk somewhat almost immediately, and it reduces it substantially within only 1 year.

Diet: It has long been known that diets low in saturated fats and high in fruits and vegetables lead to a decreased risk of heart disease. However, recent evidence also suggests that diets high in refined sugars and other carbohydrates with a high glycemic index (they cause significant increases in insulin release after ingestion) can lead to CHD. This is the basis for the popularity of The Atkins Diet and The South Beach Diet. Check with your doctor to find what the latest thinking is on diet and vascular disease at the time you buy this book.

Elevated levels of C-reactive protein: C-reactive protein (CRP) is a protein secreted by the liver in response to inflammation anywhere in the body. A high concentration of C-reactive protein in the blood (an elevated CRP level) may indicate that there is inflammation in the arteries, which can lead to atherosclerosis and CHD. C-reactive protein is now known to have direct adverse effects on capillaries as well as being involved in inflammation.

Elevated levels of plasma homocysteine: An elevated plasma level of homocysteine (hyperhomocysteinemia) has been identified as an independent risk factor for developing atherosclerosis, and subsequently CHD.

Hypertension (high blood pressure): There is a strong correlation between elevated blood pressure and CHD. It is thought that only people with a systolic blood pressure (the force of blood in the arteries as the heart beats) of 140 or greater and a diastolic pressure (the force of blood in the arteries as the heart relaxes between beats) of 90 or greater were at increased risk of developing CHD. In 2003, however, the National Heart, Lung, and Blood Institute (NHLBI) decided that if your blood pressure is between 120/80 and 139/89, then you are *prehypertensive*. This means that you don't have high blood pressure now, but are very likely to develop it in the future. Therefore, if your blood pressure falls into the prehypertensive range, don't rest on your laurels. The reality is that about 90 percent of all adults who live to be over 55 will develop hypertension eventually. Continue to have your blood pressure evaluated every year, because hypertension is treatable with medications and lifestyle changes like diet and exercise.

Obesity: The more overweight you are, the more likely you are to get CHD or have a heart attack. That's because carrying all that fat that needs to have blood pumped to it increases the heart's work. It also raises blood pressure and blood cholesterol and triglyceride levels and lowers HDL ("good") cholesterol levels. Obesity also increases the risk of getting diabetes, which will also promote CHD.

Sedentary lifestyle: Physical inactivity is a major risk factor for CHD. Studies show that even moderate exercise, like walking, reduces the risk of CHD by improving circulation, enhancing efficient use of fats and sugars, and helping to lower blood pressure and cholesterol levels.

Nonmodifiable

Age: About 85 percent of people who die of coronary heart disease are age 65 or older. (Alas, there is no way we can modify our age!)

Diabetes: CHD is the leading cause of diabetes-related death. Chronically high blood sugar is associated with narrowing of the arteries, increased blood levels of triglycerides, decreased levels of "good" HDL cholesterol, and high blood pressure. Adults with diabetes have cardiovascular death rates about two to four times higher than those of adults without diabetes.

Ethnicity: African-Americans have a greater incidence of high blood pressure than Caucasians, and consequently their risk of CHD is greater. CHD risk is also higher among Mexican Americans, American Indians, and native Hawaiians. This is partly due to higher rates of obesity and diabetes among these groups.

Gender: Overall, men have a greater risk of heart attack than women, and they have attacks earlier in life. Even after menopause, when the women's death rate from heart disease increases, it's not as great as men's until both groups are over age 80.

Family history: A family history of CHD in parents or siblings is a major risk factor for this disease. The more family members affected, the higher your risk.

Hereditary hemochromatosis: Hemochromatosis is an overload of iron in the body. Excess iron is deposited in the cells of the liver, heart, pancreas, joints, and pituitary gland. This excess is now known to cause many diseases, including heart disease, liver cancer, cirrhosis, diabetes, arthritis, and general decreased life expectancy. In hereditary hemochromatosis, the iron buildup is the result of a genetic defect that predisposes an individual to absorbing far too much iron from their diet.

Your Risk Level

When assessing the risk of CHD, it is important to remember that the greater the number and severity of risk factors, the greater is your overall risk.

Risk Factor	Number of Points
Smoker: 10–20 pack-years	2
Smoker: more than 20 pack-years	4
Obese	2
Male	2
Sedentary lifestyle	2
Over 60 years of age	2
Longtime diabetic (longer than 15 years)	4
Single first-degree relative diagnosed with CHD	4
Two or more first-degree relatives diagnosed with CHD	8
Total cholesterol over 240	2
HDL cholesterol less than 40	2
LDL cholesterol greater than 150	2
Triglycerides over 150 mg/dl	2
Elevated plasma CRP	2
Elevated plasma homocysteine	2

Total Points	Lifetime Risk of CHD
0–4	Low
5–8	Moderate
9 or more	High

Tests You May Want to Request

Luckily, there are a number of tests available to determine the status of your coronary arteries and your risk for CHD. If you are concerned about your risk factors for coronary heart disease, you should turn to these chapters: Blood Glucose Tests for Type 2 Diabetes, on page 146; Blood Tests for Hemochromatosis, on page 149; EBCT for Coronary Heart Disease, on page 177; ITST for Carotid Heart Disease, on page 199; C-Reactive Protein and Homocysteine Tests for Coronary Heart Disease Risk, on pages 159 and 197.

Read these chapters carefully so that you can decide which tests to request at your next checkup.

ESOPHAGEAL CANCER AND BARRETT'S ESOPHAGUS

The esophagus is a tube about 10 to 16 inches in length that is part of the digestive tract. It is located behind the trachea, which is the tube going to the lungs. The major function of the esophagus is to carry food from the mouth to the stomach. During the process of swallowing, circular muscles in the esophagus squeeze in an orderly fashion to propel the food toward the stomach. Glandlike cells produce mucus that acts as a lubricant to facilitate movement of food through the tube.

Cancer of the esophagus is the 20th most common cancer in the United States. Annually, approximately 13,100 Americans are diagnosed with esophageal cancer, and 12,600 die of this disease, reflecting its very high mortality rate. The incidence of esophageal adenocarcinoma has risen considerably over the past 2 decades, such that it is now more prevalent than squamous cell cancer in the United States and Western Europe.

Unfortunately, esophageal cancer does not produce symptoms until it has progressed substantially, usually to the point of metastasis—when it spreads to other tissues. Because of this, only between 5 and 10 percent of patients with esophageal cancer are cured. For patients who are candidates for surgery, the cure rate can be up to 20 percent. Therefore, using a screening tool to find this disease early is the only way to increase the survival rate for this cancer.

There are two main types of esophageal cancer.

SQUAMOUS CELL CARCINOMAS

Most of the length of the esophagus is lined with squamous cells. If a cancer arises from these cells, it's called a squamous cell esophageal cancer. They account for less than half of all esophageal cancers.

ADENOCARCINOMAS

The areas at the bottom of the esophagus and where it joins the stomach are lined with columnar cells. If a cancer grows here, it's called an esophageal adenocarcinoma. They account for greater than 50 percent of all cases.

Risk Factors

MODIFIABLE

Alcohol use: Chronic or heavy use of alcohol is a major risk factor for esophageal cancer. People who use both alcohol and tobacco have an especially high risk of esophageal cancer. Scientists believe that these substances increase each other's harmful effect.

Aspirin use: Studies have found that regular aspirin use significantly decreases the risk of developing esophageal cancer.

Diet: Diets low in vegetables and fruits are associated with an increased risk of esophageal cancer.

Gastroesophageal reflux disease (GERD): A population-based case-control study suggested that symptomatic GERD is a risk factor for esophageal adenocarcinoma. The more frequent and severe the symptoms, the more risk there is of esophageal cancer. This is a modifiable risk factor—GERD can be controlled with medications and modified eating habits. If you have symptoms of GERD—burning chest pain after meals or at night, and regurgitation (burping up) of stomach acid—consult your doctor about how to control it. Many people with chronic GERD probably develop Barrett's esophagus (see below) prior to developing esophageal adenocarcinoma.

Obesity: Studies show that there is a strong relationship between obesity and adenocarcinoma of the esophagus.

Tobacco: Smoking cigarettes or using smokeless tobacco is one of the major risk factors for esophageal cancer.

Nonmodifiable

Age: Esophageal cancer is more likely to occur as people get older; most people who develop this cancer are over age 60.

Barrett's esophagus: Not all cancers offer the opportunity to find a premalignant stage, but esophageal cancer does (predominately for the adenocarcinoma form). Barrett's esophagus is typically present for several years before esophageal cancer develops.

Tissues at the bottom of the esophagus can become irritated if stomach acid frequently backs up into the esophagus—a problem called gastroesophageal reflux disease (GERD; see modifiable risk factors, above). Over time, cells in the irritated part of the esophagus can change and begin to resemble other cells that shouldn't be there. This condition may develop into an adenocarcinoma of the esophagus and is called Barrett's esophagus.

Patients with Barrett's esophagus usually have the same symptoms everyone with GERD experiences (such as heartburn and regurgitation of fluid). Heartburn is a burning sensation behind the breastbone, usually in the lower half, but which may extend all the way up to the throat. Sometimes it is accompanied by burning or pain in the pit of the stomach. Patients with GERD also tend to regurgitate a bitter tasting fluid up from their stomach. GERD symptoms are usually worse after meals and when lying on your back. Generally, Barrett's patients tend to have more severe GERD. If you have had chronic, untreated GERD for more than 10 years, you should seriously consider having an esophagogastroduodenoscopy (EGD), especially if you are a white male.

The typical patient with Barrett's esophagus is a middle-age or elderly white male with a long history of GERD. Men get Barrett's esophagus and esophageal adenocarcinoma up to seven times as often as women, and white males develop Barrett's esophagus and adenocarcinoma of the esophagus at rates three to four times higher than males of other ethnic groups.

About two million people in the United States are believed to have Barrett's esophagus, but only about 1 percent of these people will go on to develop esophageal cancer. However, Barrett's esophagus remains the highest risk factor for esophageal cancer, and it is estimated that out of the approximately 13,000 cases of esophageal cancer diagnosed yearly, up to 10,000 of these patients will have had Barrett's esophagus–related changes as a precursor.

And it is getting more worrisome. The incidence of Barrett's esophagus–related esophageal adenocarcinoma is rising faster than that of any other cancer in the United States. Barrett's-related cancers tripled between 1976 and 1990 and more than doubled in the past decade. See EGD for Esophageal Cancer and Stomach Cancer, on page 180, for more information on Barrett's esophagus.

Diagnosis of achalasia: In this disease, the lower esophagus does not relax properly to allow food and liquid to pass into the stomach. The esophagus above this narrowing becomes dilated (larger) and retains food. It is not known why achalasia is a risk factor for esophageal cancer, but roughly 6 percent of all achalasia patients will develop squamous cell esophageal cancer.

Ethnicity: Squamous cell carcinoma of the esophagus remains four to five times more likely to occur in black males than in white males. Rates generally increase with age in all ethnic groups, but this type of esophageal cancer is consistently more common in Blacks than in Whites. On the other hand, adenocarcinoma of the esophagus is three to four times more common among Caucasians.

Gender: Squamous cell carcinoma of the esophagus is about three times more common in men than in women, and adenocarcinoma of the esophagus is about seven times more prevalent in men. Of the new cases of esophageal cancer reported each year, about 9,800 occur in men and 3,300 occur in women.

Other esophageal irritation: Other causes of significant irritation or damage to the lining of the esophagus, such as swallowing lye or other caustic substances, can increase the risk of later developing esophageal cancer.

Your Risk Level

As always, the more risk factors you have, the greater your composite risk.

Risk Factor	Number of Points
Smoker: 20 pack-years	2
Smoker: 40 pack-years	4
Excessive alcohol use for more than 20 years	2
Excessive alcohol use for more than 40 years	4
Obese	1
Male	2
Between 60 and 69 years of age	2
Older than 70 years of age	3

Risk Factor	Number of Points
Diet low in vegetables and fruits	1
Long history of GERD	4
Diagnosed with achalasia	3
Diagnosed with Barrett's esophagus	7

Total Points	Lifetime Risk of Esophageal Cancer
0–4	Low
5–8	Moderate
9 or more	High

Tests You May Want to Request

A **Barium swallow** (also called an esophagram), involves drinking a liquid containing barium, which coats the inside of the esophagus. The barium makes any changes in the shape of the esophagus show up on a series of x-rays that are taken after the barium is ingested. Although a barium swallow is used to find abnormal changes in the esophagus, this is generally done only in patients with symptoms who already have a significant tumor in the esophagus, which is likely to show up on an x-ray. Also, a barium swallow is very unlikely to detect Barrett's esophagus, the precursor to esophageal adenocarcinoma.

There is essentially only one exam that can effectively diagnose Barrett's esophagus or *early* esophageal cancer, and that is an **esophagogastroduodenoscopy**, or EGD.

An EGD involves visually examining the lining of the esophagus, stomach, and upper duodenum (first part of the small intestine) with a small camera called an endoscope, which is inserted down the throat. See page 180 for more information on this test.

HEMOCHROMATOSIS AND HEREDITARY HEMOCHROMATOSIS

Hemochromatosis is an overload of iron in the body. Excess iron is deposited in the cells of the liver, heart, pancreas, joints, and pituitary gland. This excess is known to cause heart disease as well as liver cancer, cirrhosis, diabetes, arthritis, and general decreased life expectancy. In 1992, the American Heart Association published a study carried out by Finnish researchers. The researchers found that men in the study with high levels of iron had a 220 percent greater risk of having a heart attack.

Normally, dietary iron is absorbed mainly in upper parts of the small intestine. A molecule on the lining of the intestine grabs the ingested iron and carries it across the cells that line the intestine, thus allowing the iron to be absorbed into the body. After iron is absorbed from the small intestine, it is carried in the bloodstream by a special protein called transferrin. About 20 to 45 percent of the transferrin binding sites are typically filled with iron (the percent transferrin saturation). Most absorbed iron is used in bone marrow for making new red blood cells, but about 10 to 20 percent of it goes into a storage pool.

Excess dietary iron is not usually absorbed when the cells lining the small intestine have accumulated a sufficient load of iron. These cells, known as dietary regulators, block additional uptake, preventing iron overload. A malfunctioning dietary regulator is the cause of hereditary hemochromatosis (HHC) and subsequent iron overloading. People with HHC have an inherited propensity to overabsorb iron.

According to current estimates, three to eight people per 1,000 have primary HHC, which is a high incidence for a genetic disease. But roughly one in 10 Americans, or about 25 million people, have

JUST A MINUTE . . . I THOUGHT IRON WAS GOOD FOR ME!

Of course, you did. That is because everybody told you so. For nearly 6 decades, the United States Food and Drug Administration (FDA) has required food manufacturers to enrich breakfast cereals and certain other processed foods with iron. The original purpose was to eradicate iron-deficiency anemia, the most common deficiency disease in the United States. Only recently have researchers begun questioning the safety of dietary iron supplementation, at least for much of the adult population.

There is, of course, no question that iron is important and necessary for maintaining health, but a well-balanced diet contains sufficient iron to meet the body's requirements. About 10 percent of the normal 10 to 20 mg of dietary iron is absorbed each day, and this is sufficient to balance daily iron losses. When we use or lose excessive amounts of iron for particular reasons (growth in childhood, greater iron loss with minor hemorrhages, menstruation in women, and greater need for iron in pregnancy) our bodies will compensate and increase iron absorption to around 20 percent.

the single mutated gene that causes secondary HHC, a less severe form of the disease. People with both conditions absorb and store iron at levels above normal—putting them at increased risk for CHD and other diseases. In 1997, the Centers for Disease Control (CDC) in Atlanta recommended all adults be tested for HHC, stating that it was much more prevalent than previously believed.

"Most physicians whom you mention this disease to say 'That's no big deal; it's just a rare disease,'" said Sharon McDonnell, M.D., a medical epidemiologist at CDC. "They are not familiar with the more recent findings." A 2002 survey of physician knowledge in the journal *Genetic Medicine* supports her assertion, concluding, "Many physicians have inadequate knowledge about HHC diagnosis and treatment."

Risk Factors

MODIFIABLE

If you have a malfunctioning dietary regulator due to primary or secondary HHC, the following risk factors can *increase* your risk for iron overload.

Diet: A diet rich in meat, liver, seafood, or iron-fortified processed foods like cereals can increase risk.

Iron supplements: These are often part of a multivitamin.

Transfusions: Frequent blood transfusions can put you at greater risk.

NONMODIFIABLE

Ethnicity: Primary and secondary HHC is the most common genetic disorder among Caucasians, particularly those of Northern European descent. HHC is found most often in people living in countries that surround the North Sea, particularly the United

Kingdom, Ireland, Denmark, Iceland, Norway, the Netherlands, and Germany.

Family history: If either of your parents or any of your siblings have had a positive genetic test for primary or secondary HHC, you are at higher risk for having the same disorder.

Your Risk Level

Certainly, anyone with a first- or second-degree relative with primary or secondary HHC is at sufficient risk to warrant testing. And of course, anyone who is found to have hemochromatosis based on the results of the tests described below should subsequently be tested for this genetic disorder.

If you are a diabetic with other known risk factors for heart disease like high cholesterol, it would be wise to have your iron status evaluated. Even "normal" levels of total body iron can promote CHD in some diabetics.

But what if you are simply of Northern European descent, particularly of Celtic ancestry? Does that put you at sufficient risk for HHC to be tested for it?

Well, consider this recent study: Screening for primary (homozygous) HHC was offered to all employees of the Massachusetts Polaroid Corporation due to the high proportion of employees of Celtic ancestry. 2,294 employees were screened, and five cases of primary HHC were detected. All five were Caucasian men. Four of the five cases were of 100 percent British-Irish ancestry. Additional analysis revealed that the majority of grandparents of all four individuals came from Ireland or Wales.

The authors concluded that there is a significant association of primary HHC with Celtic ancestry. But most important, if this random screening had not been done, these five men would undoubtedly have gone on to suffer irreparable heart and liver damage before they were finally diagnosed! Finding out that they had primary HHC prior to developing symptoms of these diseases probably saved them from an early death.

Tests You May Want to Consider

In order to determine whether your body is overloaded with iron, there are two blood tests available: the **percent transferrin saturation** and the **serum ferritin test**. Furthermore, there is a **genetic test** to determine if you have the inherited form of hemochromatosis, HHC. All of these tests are described in more detail in Blood Tests for Hemochromatosis, on page 149.

HEPATITIS C

Viruses, bacteria, drugs, toxins, and alcohol can all cause hepatitis (damage and inflammation in the liver). The hepatitis C virus (HCV) is one of six viruses that together account for the majority of cases of hepatitis. Infection with HCV is common, and the course of the disease is highly variable, ranging from no clinical problems to cirrhosis or cancer of the liver.

If you are harboring this virus, lifestyle habits can significantly alter its course. For example, people infected with HCV who drink alcohol or continue to use intravenous drugs can exacerbate damage to the liver. Therefore, if you become aware that you are harboring the virus and subsequently adopt a healthy lifestyle (including abstaining from alcohol), the virus might never produce serious problems for you.

Estimates have shown that in the United States alone, close to 5 million people are infected with HCV, and approximately 30,000 new infections occur each year. But most important, it is estimated that only 25 to 30 percent of these infections are actually diagnosed! The other 70 to 75 percent of people infected with HCV walk around unaware that they are carrying the virus, unless symptoms develop. HCV infection causes up to 10,000 deaths in the United States each year (a number that will likely triple in the next 20 years), and is the leading cause of liver transplants in this country. Also, unlike hepatitis A and B viruses, there is currently no effective vaccine to prevent infection from HCV.

Over 200 million people around the world are infected with HCV. This makes hepatitis C one of the greatest public health threats in the world today. Many more people are infected with HCV than HIV (the virus that causes AIDS). It is believed that without swift intervention to curtail the spread of HCV, the death rate from HCV will surpass that from AIDS in the not-so-distant future.

Risk Factors

MODIFIABLE

Intravenous drug use: Most HCV infections are due to using IV drugs with contaminated needles. People who have ever injected illegal drugs, even if they only experimented a few times many years ago, are at increased risk for HCV. It is believed that intravenous drug use now accounts for about 60 percent of HCV transmission in the United States.

Sexual activity: HCV can be spread by sex, but this does not occur as commonly as it does with hepatitis B virus. About 15 percent of HCV infections are transmitted through sexual intercourse. High-risk sexual behavior associated with increased risk of getting HCV include:

• Multiple sex partners

• Sex with prostitutes

• Traumatic sex

• Sexual intercourse during menstruation

Among married couples, if one partner is infected, the other partner is at increased risk. The risk of transmission increases with the duration of the marriage. This may occur through sexual intercourse, or it could even be due to sharing of household items like razors or toothbrushes.

Tattooing and body piercing: Hepatitis C may be passed through tattooing. Reusing tattooing needles or dye, inadequate sterilization of needles between customers, or other breaks in sterile techniques can all lead to hepatitis C infection. Body piercing may also be a source of hepatitis C infection, since it involves the use of needles and possible exposure to blood.

NONMODIFIABLE

Blood transfusions: People who received a blood transfusion or solid organ transplant before July 1992 are at increased risk for HCV, because prior to this time, the blood supply was not effectively screened for HCV. People who were notified that they received blood from a donor who later tested positive for hepatitis C are, of course, also at increased risk. However, in the last 10 years, it is believed that blood transfusions account for less than 5 percent of the cases of HCV.

Born to HCV-positive mother: If your mother had HCV at the time she gave birth to you, it is possible (although not certain) that you acquired the HCV virus at that time.

Clotting factors: Hemophiliacs who received a blood product for clotting problems before July 1992 are also at increased risk for HCV infection.

Hemodialysis: People who have been on long-term kidney dialysis are at increased risk for HCV infection. The incidence of HCV infection is higher among patients in dialysis centers than the general population, because the same dialysis equipment is used for many patients. If this equipment is not adequately sterilized, there is the possibility of transmitting HCV from one patient to another.

Needlestick: Needlestick injuries commonly occur in the health care setting, when a health care worker is accidentally jabbed with a used needle. The chances of transmitting HCV through a needle-stick are thought to be greater than the chances of transmitting HIV in this manner. Anyone receiving a needlestick with blood from a patient of unknown HCV status should be tested for the HCV virus a month or two later.

Time spent in prison: The Centers for Disease Control and Prevention have stated that HCV is extremely common in America's prison system. In fact, some data indicate that the infection rate among inmates is as high as 18 percent, compared to around 1.6 percent in the general population. As of 2001, that translated into about 360,000 of the nation's two million inmates being infected with HCV. Therefore, anyone who has spent any time at all in prison should be tested for HCV.

Your Risk Level

As always, the more risk factors you have for this disease, the more compelling your reasons for being tested. However, in the case of HCV, many an individual risk factor is sufficient to warrant testing.

If you are at moderate or high risk, we recommend a blood test known as an **enzyme-linked immunosorbent assay** (ELISA) as the initial test to determine if you have been infected with HCV. Turn to page 185 for more information on this test.

Risk Factor	Number of Points
History of injected drug use	9
Sex with multiple partners	3
History of sex with prostitutes	5
Sex with an infected steady partner	9
Born to infected mother	9
Recipient of clotting factors made before 1992	9
Recipient of clotting factors made after 1992	3
Recipient of blood or solid organs before 1992	9
Recipient of blood or solid organs after 1992	3
Hemodialysis patient	3
Undiagnosed liver problems	5
Needlestick injury	5
Multiple tattoos or body piercings	3
Time spent in prison	3

Total Points	Lifetime Risk of HCV Infection
0–4	Low
5–8	Moderate
9 or more	High

HEREDITARY NONPOLYPOSIS COLORECTAL CANCER

Of all colon cancers that are diagnosed in the United States, most are sporadic, meaning that the affected person does not have a strong family history of the disease. However, up to 10 percent of colon cancers are thought to be due to an inherited gene mutation. Hereditary nonpolyposis colorectal cancer (HNPCC) is one of the forms of hereditary colorectal cancer. (For more about colorectal cancer in general, see page 62.)

Patients with the HNPCC gene mutation have an 80 percent lifetime chance of developing colorectal cancer, compared to around a 6 percent lifetime risk in the general population. HNPCC is also characterized by:

- An average age of 45 years at diagnosis of colon cancer (compared to an average age of 65 years for colon cancer in the general population)

- Tumors that are more likely to develop in that portion of the colon which cannot be examined with flexible sigmoidoscopy (but can be visualized with a full colonoscopy)

- An increased incidence of synchronous (more than one cancer occurring at the same time) and metachronous (more than one cancer occurring at different times) colon cancers

- Polyps that show a more rapid rate of change from the non-cancerous (benign) state to the cancerous (malignant) state

- Mutations in a set of genes known as mismatch repair genes

Because the inherited HNPCC gene mutation is present in every cell in the body, other organs besides the colon can develop cancers, too (although the colon is usually the most common site of malignancy). Cancer of the uterus is also very common and may be the main cancer in some HNPCC families. Other cancers can occur in the rest of the gastrointestinal tract (stomach, small intestine), urinary system (kidneys, ureter), and female reproductive organs (particularly the ovaries).

The most critical fact is this: The vast majority of individuals with HNPCC develop *some* form of cancer.

There are at least five gene mutations that, if inherited, cause HNPCC. These five genes are called mismatch repair genes (MMR genes) because they are normally responsible for repairing mistakes in our DNA sequence each time a cell replicates itself. When they are damaged or mutated, they fail to do their job, and cell growth can become uncontrolled, so the risk of cancer increases.

People with HNPCC have a 50 percent chance of passing the faulty HNPCC gene or genes to each of their children. Some individuals with the HNPCC mutation do not have an affected parent; these individuals, who are the first to have the condition, are referred to as having a new mutation (newly altered gene). They can, however, pass this newly mutated gene to their children.

Risk Factors

Because this is a genetic condition, we do not list modifiable risk factors here—you either have the gene(s) or you don't, and your family history will be the primary determinant as to whether you should be tested. Doctors typically use criteria known as the Amsterdam II criteria to determine a person's risk for carrying the gene mutations that produce HNPCC.

- You have at least three relatives with an HNPCC-associated cancer (colorectal cancer, cancer of the endometrium, small bowel, ureter, or kidney).
- One of these relatives is a first-degree relative of the other two.
- At least one was diagnosed before age 50.
- At least two generations of your family were affected.
- Familial adenomatous polyposis (another inherited condition

WHY DO I NEED TO KNOW IF I HAVE AN MMR MUTATION?

Even if you've already been diagnosed with colorectal cancer, the presence of MMR gene mutations puts you at additional risk for other cancers. If you are aware of your higher risk, you can take measures to reduce your risk of incurring those other cancers.

Also, finding these genetic mutations has deeply important implications for your relatives—your children and siblings in particular. This information will help them determine if they, too, should be tested for these mutations.

If you already have been diagnosed with colorectal cancer, you are most likely to have MMR genetic mutations for HNPCC if your tumor tested positive for microsatellite instability. If so, you would then be a candidate for genetic testing to see if you actually have one of the common MMR gene mutations.

that can lead to colorectal cancer) is not involved for any of the cancer cases.

• Tumors were verified by pathological examination.

Approximately half of all people who meet all of the above criteria turn out to have detectable mutations in their MMR genes. Information about **HNPCC genetic testing** is found on page 192.

Risk of Cancer Due to an MMR Gene Mutation

Colon cancer risk: Patients with the HNPCC gene mutation have an 80 percent lifetime chance of developing colorectal cancer, compared to 6 percent in the general population.

Ovarian cancer risk: The risk of ovarian cancer associated with mutations in the MMR genes causing HNPCC is approximately 9 percent, which is substantially higher than the general population risk of around 1.8 percent.

Uterine cancer risk: Women who carry mutations in MMR genes have a significantly increased lifetime risk for developing uterine cancer, which may be as high as 60 percent.

Stomach, small intestine, ureter, and renal pelvis cancer risk: In people with the HNPCC gene mutation, the lifetime risk of stomach, ureter, and renal pelvis cancer runs around 10 to 20 percent, while the lifetime risk of cancer of the small intestine is around 1 to 5 percent.

HIV AND AIDS

AIDS (Acquired Immune Deficiency Syndrome) was first recognized in 1981. The first reported symptoms of AIDS were an unusual type of pneumonia and rare skin tumors. The patients were noted to have a severely low number of a specific type of immune blood cells, called the CD4+ (helper) T-lymphocycte cells. Since these cells play a critical role in helping the body fight infections, patients were susceptible to many types of infections and certain cancers.

In 1984, researchers discovered the primary viral agent of AIDS, the human immunodeficiency virus type 1 (HIV-1). In 1986, a second type of HIV, called HIV-2, was isolated from AIDS patients in West Africa. Both HIV-1 and HIV-2 have the same modes of transmission and are associated with similar infections and with AIDS. People who are infected with HIV-2 have milder, more slowly developing immunodeficiency. Nearly all cases of HIV infection in the United States are due to HIV-1. As reports of HIV-2 infection are rare, the term "HIV" used throughout this chapter will refer only to HIV-1.

Between 1992 and 1999, the number of people living with AIDS increased as a result of the continued spread of the virus and an improved survival rate. Since 1985, the proportion of all AIDS

HIV POSITIVE VERSUS AIDS

HIV, the human immunodeficiency virus, is the virus that causes AIDS. AIDS is the name given for the susceptibility to a variety of diseases that are caused by HIV infection.

The United States Centers for Disease Control (CDC) has compiled a list of all the infections and tumors that doctors use to define a person as having AIDS. If a person with HIV develops tuberculosis, for example, he or she is then said to have developed AIDS. The same is true for various other infections. A CD4+ T-cell count below 200 cells per microliter of blood is yet another sign of AIDS. You could say that AIDS is the disease and HIV is the cause of the disease.

cases reported among adult and adolescent women has more than tripled, from 7 percent in 1985 to 25 percent in 1999.

The epidemic has increased most dramatically among women of color. African-American and Hispanic women together represent less than one-fourth of all United States women, yet they account for more than three-fourths (78 percent) of AIDS cases among women.

HIV is present in the blood and genital secretions of virtually all infected individuals, regardless of whether or not they have symptoms. The spread of HIV can occur when these secretions come in contact with tissues such as those lining the vagina, anal area, mouth, or eyes (the mucosal membranes), or with a break in the skin, such as from a cut or puncture by a needle. The most common ways in which HIV is spreading throughout the world include sexual contact, needle sharing, and transmission from infected mothers to their newborns during pregnancy, labor (the delivery process), or breastfeeding.

DOES HIV ALWAYS LEAD TO AIDS?

Possibly, but this is not known with absolute certainty. About half of the people with HIV develop AIDS within 10 years, but the time between infection with HIV and the onset of AIDS can vary greatly. The severity of the HIV-related illness or illnesses will differ from person to person, according to many factors, including overall health and the medications being used to control the virus. Since the latest medications have become available for people who are HIV positive, it is possible that some of the people taking these medicines as prescribed might never go on to develop full-blown AIDS.

Risk Factors

MODIFIABLE

Intravenous drug use: Since the HIV epidemic began, injection drug use (IDU) has directly and indirectly accounted for more than one-third (36 percent) of AIDS cases in the United States alone. This disturbing trend appears to be continuing. Of the 42,156 new cases of AIDS reported in 2000, 11,635 (28 percent) were IDU-associated. A recent study showed that HIV can survive in a used syringe for at least 4 weeks. People who have sex with an injection drug user also are at higher risk for infection.

Sexual activity: The highest risk sexual activity that results in AIDS infection is thought to be anal intercourse without a condom. In this case, the risk of infection may be as high as 3 to 5 percent for each exposure. It is important to recognize, however, that HIV infection can occur after any sexual event.

Tattooing and body piercing. The risk of HIV transmission due to body piercing or tattoos is still unknown, and no cases have been recorded to our knowledge. Although HIV transmission is unlikely and there have been no confirmed cases, the CDC maintains that "a risk of HIV transmission does exist if instruments contaminated with blood are either not sterilized or disinfected or are used inappropriately between clients."

NONMODIFIABLE

Blood transfusions: Anyone who had a blood transfusion between 1978 and 1985 is at increased risk for HIV infection. Since 1985 all donated blood has been tested for evidence of HIV, and if found, the blood is discarded. Currently in the United States, there is only a very small chance of infection with HIV this way.

Born to HIV-positive mother: Mother-to-child transmission of AIDS varies between 14 and 39 percent of births. Studies have shown, however, that the number of infected infants could be greatly reduced if mothers used antiretroviral drugs (see "Antiretroviral Therapy," on page 235) during pregnancy and possibly even during breastfeeding after birth. In many of these cases, transmission occurred because the mother did not know she was HIV positive.

When antiretroviral drugs are used during pregnancy, the rate of mother-to-child transmission drops to less than 5 percent. Caesarian section also decreases the rate of HIV infection, suggesting that the majority of infections occur during delivery. Therefore, women at high risk who are pregnant or are planning to become pregnant should be tested for HIV infection.

Clotting factors: Anyone who received clotting factors between 1978 and 1987 is at increased risk for HIV infection. By 1985, about 10,000 hemophiliacs—about 70 percent of the hemophiliac population in the United States at the time—were infected with HIV through blood-clotting factors. Since 1987, steps have been taken to make blood supplies safer. Clotting factors are now heat treated to reduce the likelihood of transmission of HIV.

Your Risk Level

As always, the more risk factors you have for this disease, the more compelling your reasons for being tested. However, with HCV, many an individual risk factor is sufficient to warrant testing.

Risk Factor	Number of Points
Any incidence of unprotected sex with anyone who is known to have an HIV infection	5
Any incidence of unprotected anal sex with anyone who is known to have an HIV infection	8
Unprotected sex with an HIV-infected steady partner	9
Unprotected sex with multiple partners since 1978	4
History of sex with prostitutes	5
History of intravenous drug use	9
Born to an infected and untreated mother	9
Born to an infected but treated mother	5
Recipient of clotting factors made before 1987	9
Recipient of clotting factors made after 1987	3
Recipient of blood or solid organs before 1985	9
Recipient of blood or solid organs after 1985	3
Needlestick injury	4
Multiple tattoos or body piercings	3

Total Points	Lifetime Risk of HIV Infection
0–4	Low
5–8	Moderate
9 or more	High

Available Screening Tests

Fifteen years ago, we had essentially the same **antibody tests** and **plasma viral load tests** available for HIV testing that we do now—the difference is, nobody wanted to have the test done, because a positive result was essentially a death sentence. We included a chapter in this book for HIV testing because HIV is no longer as sinister a diagnosis as it was 10 or 15 years ago. With the newer medications and treatment protocols for those people found to be HIV positive, greatly extended life expectancies are now possible.

But there is an important distinction to be made here. Being HIV positive simply means that at some point you have been exposed to the virus that causes AIDS. Having AIDS, on the other hand, means that you were infected with the HIV virus, you have progressed to where you have a CD4+ T-cell count below 200 cells per microliter of blood, and you have started acquiring opportunistic infections, like tuberculosis or *Pneumocystis carinii* (*P. carinii*).

The goal in HIV testing is to find out that you have the virus *long before* you progress to the point that you actually have AIDS. Therefore, if you seem perfectly healthy but have some of the risk factors for HIV exposure, you would be doing yourself a great service to be tested for the presence of HIV (see Blood Tests for HIV, on page 151). If you have it, you can begin the therapies that are most likely to keep you healthy for many years to come. Don't wait until you are already sick to find out you are infected!

KIDNEY CANCER

Kidney cancer, also known as renal cancer, is an abnormal, uncontrolled growth of cells in the kidney. In its early stages, kidney cancer usually causes no obvious signs or symptoms. As it grows, it may invade organs such as the liver, colon, or pancreas. Kidney cancer cells may also spread (or metastasize) to other parts of the body, such as the lymph nodes, bones, or lungs.

There are four basic types of kidney tumors. In order from common to rare, they are: clear cell; papillary tumors; chromophobe tumors; and oncocytomas. Like most other cancers, kidney cancer can be hereditary as well as nonhereditary (sporadic). The sporadic type tends to form single tumors in one kidney and usually occurs in patients age 40 to 60 years, while inherited kidney cancer tends to produce multiple tumors, often in both kidneys, and has an earlier age of onset.

Kidney cancer affects roughly three out of every 10,000 people overall, and accounts for 2 to 3 percent of all cancers in adults. In 2002, about 30,000 people were diagnosed with this disease, and one-quarter to one-third of them had metastatic disease when they were diagnosed and were thus incurable. Kidney cancer is the eighth most common cancer in men and the 10th most common cancer in women.

Risk Factors

MODIFIABLE

Occupational exposure: A number of studies have examined occupational exposures to see if they increase workers' chances of developing kidney cancer. Some have found that coke oven workers in steel plants have above-average rates of kidney cancer. There is also some evidence that asbestos in the workplace may be associated with kidney cancer as well as lung cancer. Exposure to cadmium (a type of metal), and organic solvents, particularly trichloroethylene, increases the risk of kidney cancer.

Obesity: Some studies have shown an association between obesity and kidney cancer in women. One report suggests that being overweight may be a risk factor for men, too.

Radiation: Women who have been treated with radiation therapy for disorders of the uterus have a slightly higher risk of developing kidney cancer.

Smoking: Research shows that smokers are twice as likely to develop kidney cancer as nonsmokers. The longer a person smokes, the higher the risk. The risk of kidney cancer does decrease, though, for those who quit smoking.

NONMODIFIABLE

Age: One of the clear risk factors of kidney cancer is age. The cancer occurs most often between the ages of 40 and 70.

Ethnicity: Kidney cancer is somewhat more common among African American men than Caucasian men.

Family history: Most cases of kidney cancer seem to be random or sporadic. Only about 5 to 10 percent of all cases of kidney cancer are thought to have a strong genetic component. However, when kidney cancer does run in families, it is usually found in several members of the family, and the average age when diagnosed is about 40—10 to 15 years earlier than the average age at diagnosis for sporadic kidney cancer. Having one or more first-degree relatives (father, mother, brother, or sister) with kidney cancer definitely puts you at higher risk for the disease, and the more members affected, the higher your risk.

Gender: Another clear risk factor is being male, as renal cancer occurs almost twice as frequently in men as in women.

History of using pain killers: A 1999 study in the *British Journal of Cancer* suggested that heavy use of aspirin and acetaminophen slightly increases the risk of developing kidney cancer. However, this study found that people who took just one regular-strength aspirin a day for cardiovascular disease prevention were not at an increased risk.

Other diseases: There are at least two rare conditions (von Hippel-Lindau disease and Birt-Hogg-Dube Syndrome) associated with an increased risk of developing kidney cancer. Anyone who has been diagnosed with either of these diseases should have their kidneys monitored closely even though they account for less than 5 percent of all kidney cancers.

Your Risk Level

You can decide whether to ask your doctor for early kidney cancer screening testing by consulting the chart.

Risk Factor	Number of Points
Von Hippel-Lindau disease	9
Birt-Hogg-Dube Syndrome	9
Smoker: 10–20 pack-years	2
Smoker: more than 20 pack-years	4
Between ages 40 and 50	1

Risk Factor	Number of Points
Between ages 51 and 60	2
Older than 60 years of age	3
Male	2
African American	1
Single first-degree relative diagnosed after age 60	1
Two or more first-degree relatives diagnosed after age 60	3
Single first-degree relative diagnosed before age 45	3
Two or more first-degree relatives diagnosed before age 45	5
Known significant exposure to cadmium, asbestos, or organic solvents	3
Obese	1

Total Points	Lifetime Risk of Renal Cell Cancer
0–4	Low
5–8	Moderate
9 or more	High

Tests You May Want to Consider

There are a number of tests available to screen for early kidney cancer, including the **abdominal CT scan, magnetic resonance imaging** (MRI), and **intravenous pyelogram** (IVP). Due to their high cost and inconvenience, we don't recommend any of these tests as the first screening tests for kidney cancer.

Instead, we recommend the **abdominal ultrasound**—a safe, effective, and inexpensive test. See page 143 for more information on this test.

LUNG CANCER

Lung cancer is the single largest cause of cancer deaths in the United States (28 percent of all cancer deaths). Before cigarettes became popular in the beginning of the 20th century, lung cancer was considered a rare medical phenomenon. In 2001, lung cancer struck 169,500 people in the United States alone, and about 157,400 people died from it. The disease usually appears in people over 50 years old; its incidence is dropping in men, but lung cancer deaths in women have increased by a whopping 600 percent between 1950 and 2000. This is likely due to the fact that more women started to smoke from the 1940s onward. Lung cancer now accounts for a quarter of all cancer deaths in women.

Among the cancers where very little progress has been made in treatment, lung cancer stands at the very top of the list. In spite of advances in surgical techniques, chemotherapy, and radiation therapy, the average 5-year survival rate for non–small cell lung cancer has only increased from 14.5 percent to 16.3 percent in 20 years—hardly a success story. If the cancer is diagnosed when still localized (which currently only happens 19 percent of the time), the 5-year survival rate is as high as 83 percent. Early detection for this cancer is essential! Two major types of lung cancer account for more than 90 percent of all cases: small cell lung cancer (SCLC) and non–small cell lung cancer (NSCLC). SCLC is the most aggressive type of lung tumor, with average survival from diagnosis of only 2 to 4 months. Compared with other types of lung cancer, SCLC has a greater tendency to be widely spread by the time of diagnosis, but luckily, it is more responsive to chemotherapy and irradiation.

NSCLC is an aggregate of at least three distinct types of lung cancer, including squamous carcinoma, adenocarcinoma, and large cell carcinoma. These cell types are often classified together because when they haven't spread (are localized), all have the potential for cure with surgery. When the cancer is advanced, chemotherapy can relieve symptoms for a short time, but cure is seen in only a small minority.

Risk Factors

MODIFIABLE

Environmental tobacco smoke: The chance of developing lung cancer is increased by exposure to someone else's smoke. This exposure to environmental tobacco smoke is also referred to as secondhand smoke or involuntary or passive smoking.

Radon: Radon is an invisible, odorless, and tasteless radioactive gas that occurs naturally in soil and rocks. It can cause damage to the lungs that may lead to lung cancer. People who work in mines may be exposed to radon and, in some parts of the country, radon is found in houses. Your state environmental agency can provide you with radon test kits to find out if an elevated amount of radon is present in your home. If it is, steps can be taken to lower radon levels.

Smoking: Smoking cigarettes causes lung cancer. So does pipe and cigar smoking. In fact, all types of smoking combined account for about 87 percent of all lung cancers. About 15 percent of all people who smoke will develop lung cancer, with the risk varying depending on the number of pack-years. A pack-year equals the

THE DANGERS OF SMOKING

Physicians define a "significant smoker" as someone who has at least 20 pack-years of smoking history. This would equate to one pack per day for 20 years or two packs per day for 10 years. A significant smoker only has a 10 to 15 percent chance, at most, of developing lung cancer. This means that 85 to 90 percent of heavy smokers will not develop lung cancer. They are still, however, at very high risk for other diseases like emphysema, chronic obstructive pulmonary disease (COPD), peripheral vascular disease, and accelerated CHD.

number of packs of cigarettes smoked per day multiplied by the number of years that the person has smoked.

Stopping smoking greatly reduces a person's risk for developing lung cancer. Although the risk drops significantly even in the first year after quitting, an elevated risk for lung cancer can persist for more than 20 years.

NONMODIFIABLE

Ethnicity: Lung cancers account for 25 percent of all cancers diagnosed in African-American men, which is almost double the rate of the overall United States population. The lung cancer mortality rate for African-American men in the 1990s was over 46 percent higher than that of white men. Lung cancer death rates among African-American women are 20 percent higher than among white women.

Lung diseases: Certain lung diseases, such as tuberculosis (TB), increase a person's chance of developing lung cancer. The cancer tends to develop in areas of the lung that are scarred from TB.

Past exposure to asbestos: Asbestos is the name of a group of minerals that occur naturally as fibers and are used in certain industries. Asbestos fibers tend to break easily into particles that can float in the air and stick to clothes. When the particles are inhaled, they can lodge in the lungs, damaging cells and increasing the risk for lung cancer. Studies have shown that workers who have been exposed to large amounts of asbestos have a risk of developing lung cancer that is three to four times greater than that of workers who have not been exposed.

Personal history: A person who has had lung cancer once is more likely to develop a second lung cancer than a person who has never had lung cancer.

Pollution: Research has shown a link between lung cancer and exposure to certain air pollutants, such as by-products of the combustion of diesel and other fossil fuels. However, this relationship has not been clearly defined, and more research is being done.

Your Risk Level

Although there is evidence that exposure to radon, asbestos, and environmental smoke can cause lung cancer, cigarette smoking is by far the greatest risk factor for lung cancer. There is a significant relationship between the number of pack-years smoked and lung cancer risk; that is, the more you smoke cigarettes and the longer you smoke, the greater the risk of lung cancer.

It is important to understand that more than 10 years may pass before a normal cell transforms to a malignant cancer cell. Consequently, the risk of developing lung cancer can persist for over a decade after an individual stops smoking.

According to the National Cancer Institute, quitting smoking will definitively reduce the risk of death from lung cancer. After 10 years of smoking cessation, the risk of lung cancer death among former smokers is about 50 percent the risk of continuing smokers.

Risk Factor	Number of Points
Smoker: 20 pack-years or more	7
Smoker: 10–20 pack-years	6
Smoker: less than 10 pack-years	5
Past smoker: quit less than 10 years ago	4
Past smoker: quit 10–20 years ago	3
Past smoker: quit more than 20 years ago	2
Between 41 and 50 years of age	1
Between 51 and 60 years of age	2
61 years of age or older	3

Total Points	Lifetime Risk of Lung Cancer
0–4	Low
5–8	Moderate
9 or more	High

Tests You May Want to Request

There are a number of tests available to check for lung tumors, including **chest x-ray**, **sputum cytology**, and **low-dose spiral CT scan**.

The chest x-ray is not accurate enough to be used in routine screening of asymptomatic persons. A nodule has to be approximately 1 cubic centimeter in size for a chest x-ray to detect it. Unfortunately, by that time the cancer has often spread, making the disease incurable. Sputum cytology is even less effective, finding cancers only 10 to 20 percent of the time.

Fortunately, the new low-dose spiral CT scan has shown promise in detecting lung cancer when it is still in its earliest stages—and thus is still treatable. See page 203 for more information on this test.

OSTEOPOROSIS

Osteoporosis literally means porous bone. It is a disease characterized by reduced bone strength, leading to an increase in the risk of fractures. Osteoporosis is typically the result of bone loss, but a person who fails to develop optimal bone mass during childhood can also develop the condition.

Although the process of bone loss begins gradually for most people when they are in their mid- to late 30s, the process is so slow that it may take many years before it becomes critical. In women, the process can accelerate following menopause, when they experience a rapid decrease in estrogen production, which in turn leads to the loss of bone mass. *Osteopenia* is also characterized by a thinning of the bones, but less than is seen with osteoporosis—it is the precursor to osteoporosis.

Osteoporosis is often called a silent disease, because symptoms are not apparent until there is significant loss of bone density. The first sign is when the bone has become so thin that it breaks or collapses. Thus, the first symptom of osteoporosis that men and women in their 50s, 60s or 70s experience is very often an unexpected and painful fracture, usually in the wrist, spine, or hip. Occasionally, a woman might begin to lose height or develop a hunched back (dowager's hump).

Osteoporotic fractures can lead to significant pain and disability. Although a fracture of the wrist often will heal with little residual deformity, a patient may not make a complete recovery from a fractured hip or spine. The resulting disability may affect the ability to work and exercise. It may be so severe that an individual is unable to care properly for herself, leading her to become dependent upon family members or community caregivers.

Recent statistics from the National Osteoporosis Foundation estimate that more than 10 million men and women in the United States have osteoporosis, and nearly 19 million more have low bone mass, placing them at increased risk for osteoporosis and fractures. The National Institutes of Health also provides the following facts about osteoporosis and the resultant bone fractures.

- One out of every two women and one in eight men over 50 will have an osteoporosis-related fracture in their lifetime. Osteoporosis is responsible for more than 1.5 million fractures annually, including approximately 300,000 hip fractures, 700,000 vertebral fractures, 250,000 wrist fractures, and more than 300,000 fractures at other sites.

- Approximately one in five women over age 65 will sustain a hip fracture in her lifetime. Many will need to be placed in nursing homes after breaking their hips, as they will no longer be able to care for themselves.

- Each year, 80,000 men suffer a hip fracture and one-third of these men die within a year.

- It is estimated that direct expenditures (hospitals and nursing homes) for osteoporosis are $14 billion each year.

Risk Factors

MODIFIABLE

Cigarette smoking: Women who smoke have lower levels of estrogen compared to nonsmokers and frequently go through menopause earlier. Postmenopausal women who smoke may require higher doses of hormone replacement therapy to prevent osteoporosis and may have more side effects. Smokers also may absorb less calcium from their diets.

Diet: A diet chronically low in calcium and vitamin D will increase the risk of developing osteoporosis.

Excessive caffeine intake: Caffeine has long been known to accelerate bone loss in some people. Recent studies have suggested that in postmenopausal women in particular, drinking more than two or three cups of coffee daily can accelerate bone loss.

Excessive use of alcohol: Regular consumption of 2 to 3 ounces a day of alcohol may be damaging to the skeleton, even in young women and men. Those who drink heavily are more prone to bone loss and fractures, both because of poor nutrition and an increased risk of falling.

Exercise: A sedentary lifestyle increases the risk of osteoporosis. Bone is living tissue that responds to exercise by becoming stronger. The best exercise for your bones is weight-bearing exercise. These exercises include walking, hiking, jogging, stair-climbing, and weight training.

Sex hormones: Absence of normal menstrual periods (amenorrhea) in young women can result in osteopenia or osteoporosis. This is common in certain female athletes. Low testosterone levels in men can also increase the risk of osteopenia and osteoporosis. As already noted, decreased estrogen levels in postmenopausal females is a significant contributor to osteoporosis.

NONMODIFIABLE

Age: The older you are, the greater your risk of osteoporosis. Your bones become weaker and less dense as you age.

Body size: Small women with thin bones are at greater risk.

Ethnicity: Caucasian and Asian women are at highest risk. In fact, about 75 percent of the hip fractures associated with osteoporosis occur in white, postmenopausal females. African American and Latino women have a lower but still significant risk.

Family history: People whose parents have a history of osteoporotic fractures also seem to have reduced bone mass and may be at above-average risk for fractures.

Gender: Of the 29 million Americans threatened by osteoporosis annually, about 80 percent are women. After menopause, almost all women are at increased risk of osteoporosis, largely because of the rapid estrogen loss that occurs at menopause.

Medication use: Children and adolescents who use glucocorticoid steroids chronically (for conditions like asthma, cystic fibrosis, celiac disease, or inflammatory bowel disease) are at increased risk for skeletal problems. These drugs can interfere with bone modeling and result in osteoporosis or osteopenia.

Drugs used to treat seizures (such as phenytoin or gonadotropin releasing hormone analogs) can exacerbate bone loss, as can excessive use of aluminum-containing antacids and excessive levels of thyroid hormone.

There is also accumulating evidence that chronic use of the antiretroviral drugs used in the treatment of HIV infection can produce both osteopenia and osteoporosis.

Your Risk Level

The American College of Rheumatology, the National Osteoporosis Foundation, and various insurance payers have identified clinical indicators of high risk for osteoporosis. We think anyone over the age of 50 with *two or more* of these risk factors should consider baseline testing for the presence of osteoporosis.

- Women at or after menopause
- Women who have undergone removal of the ovaries
- Women and men with a family history of osteoporosis
- Young female athletes with a long history of too few menstrual cycles or no menstrual cycles associated with intense exercise

(Moderate exercise that does not affect menstrual cycles helps prevent osteoporosis.)

- Anyone who suffers from anorexia nervosa
- Anyone with x-ray evidence of osteoporosis
- Anyone with a history of fractures that occurred with essentially no trauma, called spontaneous fractures
- People with a history of rheumatoid arthritis or ankylosing spondylitis of over 5-year duration
- People with evidence of osteomalacia (soft bones)
- Anyone who has had long-term glucocorticoid steroid therapy
- Anyone who has had a loss of height of greater than 1.5 inches
- People who suffer from primary hyperparathyroidism
- Men with known testicular hypofunction (resulting in low testosterone levels)
- People with chronic kidney disease with a creatinine clearance that is less than 50 milliliters per minute
- People who have used Dilantin or Phenobarbital for over 5 years
- People who have used thyroid replacement therapy for 10 years or more
- People who are HIV positive and use antiretroviral drugs (See "HIV-Positive Individuals—Treatment Options" on page 235.)

Tests You May Want to Request

There are quite a few tests available for measuring bone mass, including the **quantitative computerized tomography** (QCT), **quantitative ultrasound** (QUS), **peripheral quantitative computerized tomography** (pQCT), **radiographic absorptiometry** (RA), and the **dual energy x-ray absorptiometry** (DEXA).

Of all of them, we recommend the DEXA, as it's the most accurate test available for diagnosing osteoporosis. See page 172 for more information on the DEXA scan.

OVARIAN CANCER

There are many types of tumors that can start in the ovaries. Some are noncancerous and can be treated with surgery. Some are cancerous, or malignant. The treatment options and the outcome for the patient depend on the type of ovarian cancer and how far it has spread before it is diagnosed.

Ovarian tumors are named according to the type of cells where the tumor originates and whether the tumor is benign or cancerous. There are three main types of ovarian tumors.

Germ Cell Tumors

Ovarian germ cell tumors develop from the cells that produce the eggs. Most germ cell tumors are benign, although some are cancerous and may be life threatening. Germ cell malignancies occur most often in teenagers and women in their twenties. Today, 90 percent of patients with ovarian germ cell tumors can be cured and fertility preserved with chemotherapy.

Stromal Tumors

Ovarian stromal tumors develop from the connective tissue cells that hold the ovary together and from the cells that produce female hormones. These tumors are quite rare and are usually not malignant.

EPITHELIAL TUMORS

Epithelial ovarian tumors develop from the cells that cover the outer surface of the ovary. Most epithelial ovarian tumors are benign; however, cancerous epithelial tumors (epithelial ovarian carcinomas or EOCs) are the most common and most deadly of all types of ovarian cancers. Overall, EOCs account for 85 to 90 percent of all cancers of the ovaries.

The stage of an EOC describes how far it has spread from its origin in the ovary. In Stage I, the cancer has not spread beyond the ovary. In Stage II, the cancer has spread to the pelvis. Stage III cancer has spread beyond the pelvis to the lining of the abdomen, the lymph nodes, or both. In Stage IV, the most advanced stage, the cancer has spread from the ovaries to organs outside of the abdominal cavity.

If diagnosed and treated while the cancer is in Stage I, the 5-year survival rate for ovarian cancer is 95 percent. Unfortunately, almost 70 percent of women with the common form—epithelial ovarian cancer—are not diagnosed until the disease is advanced to the most advanced stage, Stage IV.

Ovarian cancer accounts for only 4 percent of all cancers among women, but it is the fifth leading cause of cancer death among United States women and has the highest mortality rate of all gynecologic cancers. Every year, about 23,000 United States women are diagnosed with ovarian cancer and 14,000 women die from the disease.

In the absence of a family history of ovarian cancer, lifetime risk of ovarian cancer is 1 in 70. However, it is very important to recognize that around 90 percent of all ovarian cancers occur in women with few if any known risk factors!

Risk Factors

MODIFIABLE

Delayed childbirth: Having a first child after age 30 or never having children increases the risk of ovarian cancer. Having a baby prior to age 30, on the other hand, decreases the risk of ovarian cancer by around 45 percent. Subsequent pregnancies appear to decrease ovarian cancer risk by another 15 percent. This protective effect of having children is due to both the absence of menstrual cycles during pregnancy and lactation and the permanent change in estrogen responsiveness in ovarian cells.

Fertility drugs: A collaborative ovarian cancer study analyzed data from approximately 2,200 ovarian cancer patients and about 8,900 controls in 12 United States case-control studies. They reported that the use of fertility drugs increased a woman's risk of ovarian cancer nearly threefold and that the risk was substantially greater among women who had never had children.

Hormone replacement therapy (HRT): Researchers from the National Cancer Institute have found that women who use estrogen replacement therapy after menopause are at increased risk for ovarian cancer. Compared to postmenopausal women not using HRT, users of estrogen-only therapy had a 60 percent greater risk of developing ovarian cancer. The risk increased with length of estrogen use.

Recent long-term studies of the risk and benefits of HRT in postmenopausal women suggest that the overall risks of HRT may outweigh the potential benefits. We describe these putative risks of HRT in more detail in Breast Cancer, on page 46.

Oral contraceptive use: There is some evidence that the use of oral contraceptives *decreases* the overall risk of ovarian cancer in women. However, because oral contraceptives may slightly increase the risk of breast cancer in some women, you should discuss oral contraception and its role in ovarian cancer prevention with your gynecologist.

Tubal sterilization: Tubal sterilization reduces the risk of acquiring ovarian cancer.

NONMODIFIABLE

Age: The risk for ovarian cancer increases as a woman gets older. Before 30 years of age, the risk of developing ovarian cancer is remote and mostly limited to germ cell tumors. Even in hereditary cancer families, ovarian cancer is virtually nonexistent before age 20. Ovarian cancer incidence rises between ages 30 and 50, however, and continues to increase, although at a slower rate, thereafter. The highest incidence is found in women ages 75 to 79 years old.

BRCA1 and -2 gene mutations: Concern about family history and genetic predisposition to ovarian and breast cancers has increased since the recent identification of the BRCA1 and BRCA2 breast cancer susceptibility genes. Women who carry a defective BRCA gene may have a lifetime risk of ovarian cancer of about 20 percent. This is dramatically higher than the average woman's lifetime risk of 1.8 percent. In addition, ovarian cancer occurs an average of 20 years earlier in BRCA gene mutation carriers than it does in noncarriers.

Early menstruation or late menopause: Women who begin menstruating before age 12 or do not reach menopause until after age 50 have an increased risk for ovarian cancer. This may be because these women have more menstrual cycles throughout their lifetime.

Family history: Although reproductive, demographic, and lifestyle factors affect risk of ovarian cancer, the single greatest risk factor is a family history of the disease. A study of nearly 3,000 cases found that women with first-degree relatives who were diagnosed with ovarian cancer had almost four times the risk of women who had no affected relatives. Women with second-degree relatives with the disease had almost three times the risk.

The increased risk for women with first- and second-degree relatives with the disease is not solely attributed to defective BRCA genes. The evidence indicates that there are other genes that can mutate and produce an above-average risk of ovarian cancer. Researchers just haven't found them yet.

Your Risk Level

We have developed the following table to help women estimate their lifetime risk of acquiring ovarian cancer, based on known risk factors.

Risk Factor	Number of Points
Used HRT for over 10 years	2
Obese since childhood	2
Between 50 and 60 years of age	2
Over 60 years of age	3
Early menstruation/late menopause	2
Delayed pregnancy	2
Used fertility drugs in the past	2
Single first-degree relative diagnosed with ovarian or breast cancer	4
Two or more first-degree relatives diagnosed with ovarian or breast cancer	9
Known carrier of BRCA gene mutation(s)	9

Total Points	Lifetime Risk of Ovarian Cancer
0–4	Low
5–8	Moderate
9 or more	High

Tests You May Want to Consider

Bimanual examination involves insertion of the examiner's fingers into the vaginal vault with simultaneous palpation of the lower abdomen. Sensitivity of this test is thought to be very low due to the anatomic location of the ovaries. Cancers that are detected by pelvic examination are usually far advanced.

Abdominal ultrasonography involves the use of sound waves to map internal structures with the sound transducer placed on the abdomen. This test has limited usefulness as a screening tool for ovarian cancer because of frequent false-positive results. It is particularly unreliable in women who are obese.

The **carcinogenic antigen (CA) 125 Blood Test** measures levels of a protein that can indicate cancer if the levels are elevated. In combination with a **transvaginal ultrasound**, it can be very effective in testing for early ovarian cancer. See page 164 for more information on these tests.

Also, if your family history suggests that you may have inherited a BRCA1 or BRCA2 genetic mutation, you'll want to discuss testing with your doctor. See BRCA1 and BRCA2 Genetic Tests for Breast and Ovarian Cancer Risk, on page 155, for more information on BRCA mutations.

PANCREATIC CANCER

Like most cancers, cancer of the pancreas is not just one disease. In fact, as many as 20 different types of pancreatic tumors have been lumped under the umbrella term "cancer of the pancreas." Each of these tumors has a different appearance under a microscope. They can require different treatments, and each carries its own unique prognosis. Unlike other cancers we discuss in this book, pancreatic cancer seems to be able to spread very early on in its course. Finding pancreatic cancer at a very early stage is indeed a matter of life or death.

The pancreas is located deep in the abdomen, sandwiched between the stomach and the spine. It lies partially behind the stomach. The other part is nestled in the curve of the small intestine. To get a sense of the position of the pancreas, try this: Touch the thumb and pinkie finger of your right hand together, keeping the other three fingers together and straight. Then, place your hand in the center of your belly just below your lower ribs with your fingers pointing to the left. Your hand will be at the approximate level of your pancreas.

Because of the pancreas' deep location, tumors can rarely be felt by pressing on the abdomen. Its location also explains why many symptoms of pancreatic cancer often do not appear until the tumor grows large enough to interfere with the function of nearby structures such as the stomach, small intestine, liver, or gall-bladder. Sadly, once the tumor is this large, it is often much more difficult to treat.

Pancreatic cancer is far more common in the Western world than anywhere else, and it is an extremely deadly form of cancer. This year, approximately 29,000 Americans will be diagnosed with it, and about 98 percent of these people will eventually die from the disease. The poor long-term survival of pancreatic cancer is a result of its resistance to most treatments. This low survival rate is also due to the relatively late stage of the disease at the time of diagnosis.

The reported 5-year survival rate for pancreatic cancer that has produced no detectable sign of spreading is only 9 percent. This may not seem promising, but it is more than double the survival rate for those whose cancer has spread slightly (4 percent). If pancreatic cancer has spread throughout the body, the 5-year survival rate is a dismal 2 percent.

Fortunately, patients who have small, localized tumors that are treated and operated upon have much better 5-year survival rates. In fact, they can be as high as 37 to 38 percent. This statistic alone argues for the importance of early detection of this cancer in people who are at high risk for it. As with many other conditions, the earlier pancreatic cancer is detected, the better chance you have of recovering from the disease.

Pancreatic dysplasia is a precancerous condition that almost always precedes pancreatic cancer. The average time between the development of pancreatic dysplasia and the onset of pancreatic cancer has been reported as about 6 years. Since late detection is one of the primary reasons for the poor survival of pancreatic cancer, we believe that detecting pancreatic dysplasia offers the best opportunity for individuals at high risk for the disease to survive this deadly disease.

Risk Factors

MODIFIABLE

Cigarette smoking: Not surprisingly, smoking is the biggest modifiable risk factor for developing pancreatic cancer. For example, students who smoke cigarettes during college can have a two- to threefold increased risk of pancreatic cancer later in their lives.

Diet: Although it has been played up in the press that coffee and alcohol can cause pancreatic cancer, there is currently no strong evidence to support this statement. However, diets high in meats, fried foods, and nitrosamines (found in foods like beer, bacon, cold cuts, and other cured meats) may increase the risk of pancreatic cancer, while diets high in fruits and vegetables may reduce the risk.

Obesity: Obese men and women have an increased risk of pancreatic cancer, but that risk may be lowered by moderate physical activity, such as walking and hiking.

NONMODIFIABLE

Age: The risk of developing pancreatic cancer increases with age. Over 80 percent of the cases develop between the ages of 60 and 80.

Chronic pancreatitis: Long-term inflammation of the pancreas (pancreatitis) has been linked to cancer of the pancreas. The reason for this association is not clear, but it is greatest in patients with inherited chronic pancreatitis.

Diabetes: A number of reports have suggested that diabetics have an increased risk of developing pancreatic cancer, particularly long-standing diabetics.

Ethnicity: Pancreatic cancer is more common in the African American population than it is in the white population. Pancreatic cancer is more common in Jews—particularly Ashkenazi Jews—than the rest of the population, possibly because of the inherited mutation in the BRCA2 gene that occurs in some Jewish families (see below).

Family history: Some families have a strong history of pancreatic cancer for neither of the known genetic reasons listed above. The National Familial Pancreatic Cancer Registry (NFPTR) now contains a listing of over 250 families in which two or more family members have had pancreatic cancer.

Gender: Cancer of the pancreas is more common in men than in women.

Genetics: Johns Hopkins University has reported that as many as 10 percent of pancreatic cancers are likely caused by inherited defects in the BRCA2 gene (mutations of the gene that also increases the risk of breast and ovarian cancer). One particular defect in BRCA2 is found in about 1 percent of Ashkenazi Jews, which may explain this ethnic group's higher rate of pancreatic cancer. Testing is available for mutations in both the BRCA1 and BRCA2 genes, and is discussed in BRCA1 and BRCA2 Genetic Tests for Breast and Ovarian Cancer Risk, on page 155.

Hereditary nonpolyposis colorectal cancer (HNPCC) syndrome is characterized by the inherited predisposition to develop colon cancer, uterine cancer, stomach cancer, and ovarian cancer (see page 90). People diagnosed with HNPCC may be at increased risk for pancreatic cancer as well.

Still, the vast majority of people who acquire pancreatic cancer—around 90 percent—have no known genetic predisposition to the disease.

Your Risk Level

You can calculate your composite risk for pancreatic cancer using the table on page 124.

Risk Factor	Number of Points
Smoker: 10–20 pack-years	1
Smoker: more than 20 pack-years	3
Obese	1
Over 60 years of age	1
Diet high in meat and fried foods	1
Long time diabetic (more than 20 years)	2
History of chronic pancreatitis	3
Diagnosed with hereditary nonpolyposis colorectal cancer	2
Single first-degree relative diagnosed with pancreatic cancer	4
Two or more first-degree relatives diagnosed with pancreatic cancer	9
Known carrier of BRCA gene mutation(s)	6

Total Points	Lifetime Risk of Pancreatic Cancer
0–4	Low
5–8	Moderate
9 or more	High

Tests You May Want to Consider

Available tests include the **abdominal ultrasound**, the **CA 19-9 blood test**, endoscopic retrograde cholangiopancreatography (ERCP), and **endoscopic ultrasound** (EUS).

Abdominal ultrasound is safe and inexpensive, but there is no conclusive information on the usefulness of this test for finding pancreatic cancer or pancreatic dysplasia in people with no symptoms.

The Blood tumor marker CA19-9 test is currently used only to help in the diagnosis of pancreatic cancer in patients with symptoms and to monitor progress of the disease in patients already diagnosed with it. Among healthy, asymptomatic individuals, measuring CA19-9 alone has not been shown to be effective in detecting early disease. CA19-9 is also not considered to be useful in detecting the presence of pancreatic dysplasia.

EUS—combined with an ERCP as follow-up—is an effective screening regimen for people who are at high risk for pancreatic cancer. See page 188 for more information on these tests.

PROSTATE CANCER

The prostate is a gland found only in males. It makes and stores the milky fluid that nourishes sperm. This fluid is released along with the sperm during ejaculation to form what is known as semen. Normally, the prostate is about the size of a walnut. It is located below the bladder and in front of the rectum. It surrounds the upper part of the urethra, the tube that empties urine from the bladder. If the prostate grows too large, the flow of urine can be slowed or stopped.

Prostate cancer is the most common cancer in North American men (excluding skin cancers). It is estimated that in 2003 approximately 220,900 new cases will be diagnosed, and 28,900 prostate cancer–related deaths will occur in the United States alone. Only lung cancer kills more men than prostate cancer, which accounts for 29 percent of all male cancers and 11 percent of male cancer-related deaths.

The most common signs and symptoms of prostate cancer are:

• Weak or interrupted flow of urine

• Urinating often (especially at night)

• Difficulty urinating or holding back urine

- Pain or burning when urinating
- Blood in the urine or semen

Risk Factors

MODIFIABLE

Diet: Men who have a diet high in animal fat, red meat, and high-fat dairy products seem to have an increased risk of getting prostate cancer. Conversely, a diet high in fruits and vegetables seems to decrease the risk. Eating lots of tomatoes or tomato products (which contain large amounts of a substance called lycopene) seems to be particularly helpful in preventing prostate cancer.

Smoking: Research results regarding smoking and prostate cancer have been mixed. However, new findings published in the July 2003 issue of *Cancer Epidemiology, Biomarkers and Prevention* suggests that smoking is a significant risk factor for developing prostate cancer—particularly the deadliest forms of it. This study found that men under age 65 with a history of 40 or more pack-years (those who smoke a pack a day for 40 years or two packs a day for 20 years) face double the risk of developing more aggressive forms of prostate cancer, as compared to nonsmokers.

Vasectomy: Some studies have suggested that there may be a link between having a vasectomy and being at greater-than-average risk for developing prostate cancer. However, other studies have not supported this claim, and at present these findings are highly questionable.

NONMODIFIABLE

Age: In the United States, the risk of developing prostate cancer increases starting at age 50 in white men who have no family history of the disease, and at age 40 in African-American men who have no family history of the disease. The average age at diagnosis is about 71, and the average age of death from prostate cancer is 78. More than 75 percent of all cases of prostate cancer are diagnosed in men older than 65, and 90 percent of the deaths from this cancer occur in this age group.

Prostate cancer tends to be less aggressive when it occurs in older men than when it occurs in younger men. Since the great majority of men who get prostate cancer are over age 65, more men actually receive a diagnosis of prostate cancer in their lifetimes than die of it. In other words, when older men get it, they are more likely to die *with* prostate cancer than *from* prostate cancer.

Ethnicity: The likelihood of getting prostate cancer is approximately 60 percent higher in black men than in white men, and the mortality rate from prostate cancer is twice as high in black men as in white men. Asian American and Hispanic men have incidence rates lower than both white and black males.

Family history: Men who have a first-degree relative with prostate cancer have double the risk of developing prostate cancer during their lifetime, with increased risk starting at the age of 40. A man who has two first-degree relatives with prostate cancer has five times the chance of developing prostate cancer.

Gender: Men only, obviously.

Your Risk Level

Age (being over 50), family history (having one or more first-degree relatives with prostate cancer), and ethnicity (being African American) are each significant risk factors on their own, and any combination of them obviously puts you at even higher risk.

The American Cancer Society recommends that initial screening for prostate cancer be offered annually beginning at age 50. Men at high risk should begin testing at age 45. Men who have multiple first-degree relatives with prostate cancer should begin testing at age 40.

You can estimate your composite risk for prostate cancer using the table below.

Risk Factor	Number of Points
Between 60 and 69 years of age	3
Between 70 and 79 years of age	4
Over 80 years of age	5
Smoker: 20 pack-years	2
Smoker: 21–40 pack-years	3
Smoker: more than 40 pack-years	4
African-American	3
Diet high in red meat and animal fat	3
Vasectomy	2
Single first-degree relative diagnosed with prostate cancer over age 60	3
Single first-degree relative diagnosed with prostate cancer before age 60	5
Two or more first-degree relatives diagnosed with prostate cancer over age 60	7
Two or more first-degree relatives diagnosed with prostate cancer before age 60	9

Total Points	Lifetime Risk of Prostate Cancer
0–4	Low
5–8	Moderate
9 or more	High

Tests You May Want to Consider

Unlike most of the other diseases in this book, there is no single specific test that works best for detecting prostate cancer. There are several tests that, when looked at together, give a better prediction that the disease is or is not in fact present, compared to any single test alone. As with all other cancers, the gold standard, or real proof, for the presence of prostate cancer is a biopsy.

Digital rectal examination (DRE), using a gloved finger to feel the prostate for irregularities or lumps, is often the first test recommended. It's important to be aware, however, that this test does have a high rate of false positives.

There are blood tests available that measure the amount of **prostate specific antigen (PSA)**. If the level of this compound is elevated, it can point to possible prostate cancer. If your DRE or PSA tests indicate that you might have prostate cancer, a follow-up test called a **transrectal prostate ultrasound** may be done, in addition to a biopsy. See PSA Tests for Prostate Cancer, on page 209, for more information on these tests.

STOMACH CANCER

S tomach cancer, also called gastric cancer, is the name for cancer that begins in the stomach, generally the stomach lining. This type of cancer can eventually spread to lymph nodes and organs such as the liver, pancreas, colon, lungs, and ovaries. The stomach is a sacklike organ located just under the diaphragm, the muscle that separates the chest cavity from the abdominal cavity. (People occasionally confuse the stomach itself with the abdominal cavity, saying they have a stomachache, when really the pain could be occurring in the appendix, small intestine, colon, or gall bladder, instead of in the actual stomach itself.) The stomach has several sections, and the location of the cancer in the stomach can affect symptoms, prognosis, and treatment options.

Most stomach cancers start from the glandular cells of the stomach lining and are known as adenocarcinomas. Cancers which start from the muscle cell layer of the stomach are known as leiomyosarcomas and are a type of soft tissue sarcoma. Overall, about 50 percent of stomach cancers occur in the lower part of the stomach (the *pyloris*), 20 percent are found in the body of the stomach (*fundus*), another 20 percent are in the lesser curvature, and around 10 percent occur at the top of the stomach (*cardia*).

Stomach cancer is the seventh leading cause of cancer deaths in the United States. Doctors diagnose about 22,000 cases of new stomach cancer in the United States annually, and nearly 13,000 Americans with stomach cancer die annually. In the 1970s, it was the most common form of cancer in the world, and was highly linked to the intake of salted, smoked, and pickled foods, and infection with the *H. pylori* bacterium. Stomach cancer is less common in the United States today than it was just 40 years ago, although it remains second only to lung cancer in incidence worldwide. Part of the reason for the decline in the United States is related to changes in our diet, particularly the use of refrigeration, which has meant that people eat more fresh food and less smoked and pickled food.

Risk Factors

MODIFIABLE

Alcohol use: Heavy use of alcohol over many years is thought to increase the risk of acquiring stomach cancer.

Cigarette smoking: People who smoke have a higher-than-average risk of developing stomach cancer.

Diet: People who eat lots of salted, smoked, or poorly preserved foods and few fruits and vegetables have a higher-than-average risk of developing stomach cancer. With particular regard to salt, a 2004 study in the *British Journal of Cancer* reported that researchers from the National Cancer Center Research Institute in Japan found a link between eating even low amounts of salt and stomach cancer. These scientists found a statistically significant rise in the risk of stomach cancer for subjects who ate even 2/10 ounce of table salt per day. For those who eat 4/10 ounce of salt a day, the risk doubled.

NONMODIFIABLE

Age: Most stomach cancers occur in people over age 55.

Atrophic gastritis: There are two main types of atrophic gastritis: fundal gland (type A), and pyloric (antral) gland (type B) gastritis. These occur in older people. Antral gastritis increasingly involves the fundal gland area with advanced age.

Both types A and B are associated with intestinal metaplasia and a predisposition to gastric cancer. Type A gastritis is less common and its distribution in the stomach resembles that of pernicious anemia. Type B gastritis is predominant in those areas of the corpus where gastric cancer is common and appears to be a risk factor mainly for the intestinal type of gastric cancer. *H. pylori*, which is the cause of type B gastritis, has been implicated as a risk factor for gastric cancer.

Blood type: There is some evidence that people whose blood is Type A are more likely to get stomach cancer.

Chronic gastritis: Chronic gastritis is characterized by chronic inflammation of the gastric mucosa (lining of the stomach), which can lead to stomach ulcers. Chronic gastritis occurs most frequently in middle-age people, can lead to stomach cancer, and is often caused by a chronic *Helicobacter pylori* (*H. pylori*) bacterial infection (see below).

Note: Although people with gastritis and gastric ulcers get stomach cancer at a higher-than-average rate, this does *not* seem to be the case for people who get peptic ulcer disease (PUD), despite the fact that both disorders seem to be predominately due to *H. pylori* infection. In fact, some studies have even suggested that people with PUD are at even lower-than-average risk for developing stomach cancer.

Chronic *Helicobacter pylori* infection: *H. pylori* infection is common in the United States, with about 20 percent of people under age 40 and half of those over age 60 harboring it. This condition is a moderately strong risk factor for the development of gastric cancer, through the development of gastric atrophy and intestinal metaplasia (metaplasia is a potentially reversible change from a fully differentiated cell type to another cell type, implying adaptation to environmental changes). In the stomach, intestinal type metaplasia is most common. This often occurs as a result of *H. pylori* infection or bile reflux. Intestinal metaplasia is considered a precancerous condition.

According to The Helicobacter Foundation, *H. pylori* is classified as a grade 1 carcinogen (the same classification given to cigarette smoking). The Helicobacter Foundation reports that studies have shown *H. pylori* infection to be associated with a three to six times higher stomach cancer risk than normal and that when persons with early stomach cancer are examined, about 90 percent appear to have *H. pylori*.

Ethnicity: Stomach cancer is 1.5 to 2.5 times more common among African-Americans, Hispanics, and Native Americans than among Caucasians.

Worldwide, Japan has the highest stomach cancer incidence, closely followed by Korea. Japanese investigators have noted that more than 65 percent of Japanese above the age of 50 years are infected with *H. pylori*.

Familial adenomatous polyposis: FAP is a rare genetic condition resulting in hundreds or even thousands of polyps forming in the colon and other parts of the digestive system, leading to early colorectal cancer. Although cancer will usually develop in only the colon, polyps and cancer may also develop in the stomach in FAP.

Family history: If you have a mother, father, brother, or sister who has had stomach cancer, you have a higher-than-average risk of developing stomach cancer.

Gender: Stomach cancer affects men twice as often as women.

Hereditary nonpolyposis colorectal cancer: HNPCC occurs because of mutations in genes that are involved in DNA repair, and therefore this condition can lead to an increased risk for several types of cancer, especially colorectal cancer, but also stomach cancer (see Hereditary Nonpolyposis Colorectal Cancer, on page 90, for more information on HNPCC).

Pernicious anemia: This is an anemia (decreased oxygen-carrying ability of the blood) usually caused by the absence of intrinsic factor. Intrinsic factor is a protein that is secreted by cells of the stomach lining. Intrinsic factor attaches to vitamin B_{12} and takes it to the intestines to be absorbed into the bloodstream, where it can then go to the bone marrow and be used in the process of making red blood cells (among other things). Absence of intrinsic factor is the most common cause of pernicious anemia, and it is typically the result of an immune-related atrophy (shrinkage) of the stomach lining. This atrophy of the stomach sometimes leads to stomach cancer.

Previous stomach surgery: Partial gastrectomy for benign peptic ulcer disease is associated with an increased risk of adenocarcinoma of the stomach, especially in patients who are at least 15 years postgastrectomy.

Your Risk Level

Risk Factor	Number of Points
Smoker: 10–20 pack-years	1
Smoker: more than 20 pack-years	2
Between 50 and 60 years of age	1
Over 60 years of age	2
Chronic *H. pylori* infection	4
History of chronic gastritis	3

(continued on page 136)

Risk Factor	Number of Points
History of atrophic gastritis	3
History of pernicious anemia	2
Dietary history high in smoked, salted, and pickled foods	2
Significant history of alcohol consumption	2
Male	2
Non-Caucasian	1
Single first-degree relative with stomach cancer	4
Two or more first-degree relatives with stomach cancer	8
Gastrectomy more than 15 years ago	2
Type A blood	1

Total Points	Lifetime Risk of Stomach Cancer
0–4	Low
5–8	Moderate
9 or more	High

Tests You May Want to Request

Stomach cancer itself must be detected early in order for there to be any chance of actual cure. When the cancer has spread, the outlook is poor. The 5-year survival rate for stomach cancer is 90 percent when the cancer is detected in its earliest stages. However, most people in the United States do not receive a diagnosis until stomach cancer is more advanced. For the most advanced stage of stomach cancer, the 5-year survival rate is only 3 percent.

Fortunately, stomach cancer has premalignant changes that can be detected and then dealt with, just as is done with polyp formation in colorectal cancer, or Barrett's esophagus in esophageal cancer. The most effective tests used to find these premalignant changes is an **esophagogastroduodenoscopy** (EGD). See page 180 for more information on this test.

However, as noted above, one of the primary risk factors for acquiring stomach cancer is having a chronic *H. pylori* infection in your stomach. Therefore, most readers should have themselves **tested for chronic H. pylori infection** before considering an EGD (an exception would be someone with a strong family history of stomach cancer—get the EGD done regardless, about 5 years prior to the age of the family member who got stomach cancer at the youngest age).

Being tested for the presence of *H. pylori* is a particularly good idea if you have a history of gastroesophageal reflux disease (GERD), or have active gastric or duodenal ulcers, because *H. pylori* may be causing them (there are several drug regimens that the physician can use to eradicate the infection if it is found). See *H. Pylori* Tests for Stomach Cancer Risk, on page 191.

TYPE 2 DIABETES

Diabetes mellitus is a lifelong disease for which there is not yet a cure. It is caused by a problem in the way the body makes or uses insulin, a hormone that is produced by the pancreas. The cells of the body use glucose as an energy source, and insulin is necessary for glucose to move from the blood to the insides of the cells. Unless glucose gets into cells, the body cannot use it for energy. Therefore, if insulin fails to work properly, the amount of glucose in the blood becomes very high. Once blood glucose levels reach a high enough concentration, glucose starts to "spill over" into the urine (normally, the kidneys do not put any glucose into the urine). Glucose appearing in the urine is one of the cardinal signs of diabetes.

Type 2 diabetes is the most common form of diabetes, affecting about 90 to 95 percent of all people with diabetes. People with type 2 diabetes manufacture insulin; however, the insulin fails to work properly. Because the insulin doesn't work, glucose can't enter into cells in adequate amounts. This results in what the body perceives as an insulin deficiency, so the pancreas releases more and more insulin into the blood. The onset of this type of diabetes, also called adult-onset diabetes, or non–insulin-dependent diabetes mellitus

(NIDDM), usually occurs after age 30. About 16 million Americans have type 2 diabetes, but more important, about one-third of them are not aware of their condition. It is also a disease that is on the rise. Over the past 4 decades, there has been a sixfold increase in the number of diabetics in the United States. Much of this increase is thought to be due to the increase in obesity, and a generally more sedentary lifestyle among Americans. By 2025, there will be an estimated 300 million people with diabetes worldwide.

This is a disease that can be present for up to a decade before significant symptoms appear and it is finally diagnosed. When it is eventually diagnosed, many problems often already exist, and these problems contribute to more than 193,000 deaths each year.

Diabetes is a disease that can have devastating health effects in the long term. For example, type 2 diabetes is the leading cause of new cases of blindness in adults 20 to 74 years old. Each year, an estimated 12,000 to 24,000 people with type 2 diabetes become blind because of diabetic eye disease, and about 28,000 people develop total kidney failure. Furthermore, about 60 to 70 percent of people with type 2 diabetes have mild to severe forms of nervous system damage (which often includes impaired sensation or pain in the feet or hands, slowed digestion of food in the stomach, carpal tunnel syndrome, and other nerve problems). Severe forms of diabetic nerve disease are a major contributing cause of lower extremity amputations. People with type 2 diabetes are also two to four times more likely to develop heart disease or stroke than people without diabetes.

Risk Factors

Modifiable

Obesity: Obesity is an extremely important risk factor for developing type 2 diabetes, as over 70 percent of the people with this disease are obese. Evidence from several studies indicates that weight loss reduces the risk of developing type 2 diabetes.

Sedentary lifestyle: Even if you are not obese, people who are sedentary are much more likely to develop type 2 diabetes.

NONMODIFIABLE

Age: Most people who acquire type 2 diabetes are over age 45. However, the average age when diagnosed is dropping, probably due to more people being screened earlier for the disease.

Ethnicity: Some populations, like African-Americans, Hispanics and Native American Indians, are at greater risk of getting type 2 diabetes. About half of American Indian adults ages 45 to 74 have diabetes. The rate of diabetes has tripled for African-Americans in the past 30 years, and rates for African-American women over age 55 have reached near-epidemic proportions. In Hispanics over age 50, there is an incidence of type 2 diabetes of 25 to 30 percent.

Family history: Having one or more first-degree relatives with type 2 diabetes increases your risk of getting this disease.

Your Risk Level

Any *one* of these risk factors, whether modifiable or nonmodifiable, would warrant having the relatively inexpensive diagnostic tests for this disease.

Tests You May Want to Request

All three of the tests we recommend to check for diabetes are simple blood tests. They include the **random blood glucose level,** the **fasting blood glucose test,** and the **oral glucose tolerance test.** These tests measure the level of sugar in your blood. They are all effective for early screening for type 2 diabetes. See page 146 to determine which of them is right for you.

THREE

THE
TESTS

ABDOMINAL ULTRASOUND FOR AAA AND KIDNEY CANCER

O f all the tests available, the abdominal ultrasound is the best screening tool for abdominal aortic aneurysm (AAA) and kidney cancer in asymptomatic people. It is a very safe test, it is accurate, it involves no radiation exposure or dye injection, and it is a relatively inexpensive procedure.

Abdominal ultrasound imaging is a method of obtaining images of internal abdominal organs by sending high-frequency sound waves into the body. The reflected soundwaves' echoes are recorded and displayed as a real-time, visual image. No ionizing radiation (x-ray) is involved in ultrasound imaging. An abdominal ultrasound image is a useful way of examining internal organs, including the liver, gallbladder, spleen, pancreas, kidneys, and bladder, as well as the abdominal aorta.

Preparation for an abdominal ultrasound is very simple. You wear loose-fitting clothing and fast for at least 4 hours prior to the exam. You will be required to pull your shirt up to about 4 inches above the navel. First, a jellylike substance will be placed on your skin. Then, the ultrasound transducer will be moved over the skin on your abdomen, viewing and recording an ultrasound image. The diameter of the aorta is also measured and recorded. The procedure generally takes less than 10 minutes and is completely painless.

Reliability

AAA

Abdominal ultrasound is a very specific test for AAA, with a very low rate of false positives. Reported sensitivities are high, ranging from 82 to 99 percent, with sensitivity approaching 100 percent in some people with large AAAs. In only a small proportion of patients, factors like obesity or bowel gas will make it difficult to fully view the abdominal aorta.

KIDNEY CANCER

It has been reported that ultrasound had a detection rate of 85 percent in kidney lesions larger than 3 cm and a detection rate of less than 60 percent in lesions smaller than 2 cm. Abdominal ultrasound examination has a very high specificity (about 99 percent) and a moderate sensitivity (about 67 percent) in detecting kidney abnormalities in potential kidney donors.

A large German study published in the journal *Urologe* produced some promising evidence that abdominal ultrasound can detect kidney cancer at a stage when it is more likely to be curable. This large study compared symptomatic patients who underwent exploratory surgery with patients who underwent the same surgery because tumors were *accidentally* detected by ultrasound while the doctor was looking for something else. In other words, the latter group was asymptomatic for kidney cancer. The study showed that the tumors found "incidentally" were significantly smaller and often showed a significantly lower local tumor stage, a better tumor grade, and lymph nodes free of cancer. The renal tumors found in the asymptomatic patients also spread less frequently to other parts of the body.

Health Risks

There are no known health risks for abdominal ultrasound.

Cost

Diagnostic abdominal ultrasound is currently relatively inexpensive in the United States ($100 to $175 per examination). It is even less expensive when performed by a mobile vascular screening service, such as Life Line Screening.

BLOOD GLUCOSE TESTS
FOR TYPE 2 DIABETES

A random plasma glucose test measures the amount of glucose (sugar) in the blood at any given time. The test does not require fasting and therefore can be done at any time—even after a meal. If the amount of glucose is greater than or equal to 200 mg/dl (milligrams per deciliter), you are considered to be diabetic.

A better method for diagnosing type 2 diabetes is a **fasting blood glucose test**. It requires that you do not eat or drink anything for approximately 8 hours before the test. For this reason, it is usually done in the morning before breakfast. A normal fasting glucose level is between 70 and 110 mg/dl. A fasting glucose level between 111 and 125 mg/dl indicates some problem with glucose metabolism (you could be on your way to developing diabetes). You will be diagnosed as diabetic if your fasting glucose level is equal to or greater than 126 mg/dl.

An **oral glucose tolerance test** can be performed in a doctor's office or a lab. You'll be required to fast before this test—no food or drink for at least 10 hours before the start of the test. First, a blood glucose test is taken. Then, you'll be given a bottle of "glucola" with a high amount of sugar in it that you'll have to drink.

Your blood glucose is measured 30 minutes later, then an hour later, again after 2 hours, and finally 3 hours later.

In a person without diabetes, the blood glucose level rises immediately after drinking the glucose drink, but then falls quickly back to normal as insulin is produced. In diabetics, glucose levels rise higher than normal after drinking the glucose drink and come down to normal levels much more slowly.

A person is said to have impaired glucose tolerance when the 2-hour measurement is between 140 and 200 mg/dl. This is often referred to as prediabetes and is considered to be a risk factor for future development of diabetes.

A person actually has diabetes when the oral glucose tolerance test shows that the blood glucose level at 2 hours is 200 mg/dl or greater. This finding must then be confirmed by a second glucose tolerance test on another day.

Interpreting Your Results

People at risk for type 2 diabetes should first have a simple fasting blood glucose test. If your fasting blood glucose level is **below 110 mg/dl**, you currently do not have any problems with glucose metabolism. However, if you are at high risk for this disease, you should still have a fasting glucose done yearly.

If your fasting blood glucose is somewhere **between 111 and 125 mg/dl**, you should then have an oral glucose tolerance test as well. If your 2-hour oral glucose tolerance tests results are between 140 and 200 mg/dl, there is a high probability that you are on your way to having type 2 diabetes (that is, you are prediabetic).

If you have a fasting blood glucose level of **greater than 125 mg/dl**, you should also have an oral glucose tolerance test. If this test shows that your blood glucose level at 2 hours is 200 mg/dl or more, you already have type 2 diabetes.

If you discover you have prediabetes, you have done yourself a great service by finding out. Many studies have demonstrated that lifestyle changes alone (diet and exercise) are effective in preventing progression to type 2 diabetes.

Similarly, if you find out that you already have diabetes, you stand to benefit greatly. The Diabetes Control and Complications Trial (DCCT), first launched by the National Institute of Diabetes, Digestive and Kidney Diseases (NIDDK) in 1981, has provided dramatic evidence that early intervention in controlling blood glucose levels in diabetics greatly affects their long-term outcomes.

Conventional wisdom says that testing for diabetes or prediabetes should begin around age 45, since most type 2 diabetics are over age 45. But we believe that people at elevated risk should start having these simple, inexpensive tests beginning at age 30, to increase the likelihood of finding—and successfully treating—more prediabetics.

Reliability

All of these tests are very reliable and, because they are repeated regularly with anyone who tests positive for type 2 Diabetes, the overall accuracy approaches 100 percent.

Health Risks

There are no health risks for these tests.

Cost

A fasting blood glucose test costs between $5 and $21, and the 3-hour glucose tolerance test is between $15 and $50.

BLOOD TESTS
FOR HEMOCHROMATOSIS

The **percent transferrin saturation test (%TS)** is the preferred first screening test for hemochromatosis. It is a simple blood test that screens for the abnormal metabolism that signals a propensity to overaccumulate iron. The percent transferrin saturation test should be done after an overnight fast (at least 12 hours), and you should abstain from taking vitamin C or any iron-containing supplements for several days prior to the test.

Measuring serum ferritin levels (sFT) can also be useful in patients to detect hemochromatosis. The sFT concentration is a manifestation of an accumulation of excess iron in the body. However, a serum sFT level is not a good first test to look for HHC, because sFT can increase moderately for unrelated reasons. In addition, this test is rather expensive.

The genetic test for hereditary hemochromatosis (HHC) is performed on a blood sample. However, genetic testing for HHC should only be done after percent transferrin saturation test or sFT tests show that significant hemochromatosis is present. Going directly to genetic screening without first testing for the presence of hemochromatosis is not recommended.

Reliability

The sensitivity of the percent transferrin saturation test alone for detecting hemochromatosis is 94 to 98 percent, with a specificity of 70 to 98 percent.

The percent transferrin saturation test combined with a follow-up sFT is even more accurate.

The genetic test for HHC will detect the most common genetic mutations for HHC approximately 85 percent of the time.

Health Risks

There are no health risks for any of these tests. All three are tests that are performed on a blood sample taken during a simple blood draw.

Cost of the Screening Tests

Percent transferrin saturation testing costs between $20 and $50, and sFT generally costs around $80 to $100. Genetic testing costs between $125 and $165.

BLOOD TESTS FOR HIV

If you have any *single one* of the risk factors for HIV infection, you would be very wise to be tested for the HIV virus.

The Centers for Disease Control and Prevention (CDC) has estimated that one-fourth of the suspected 900,000 HIV-infected people in the United States are not aware that they are infected. In other words, 225,000 people in the United States have a virus in their bodies that could result in early death if left untreated to progress to full-blown AIDS.

If an HIV infection is found, and you take antiretroviral drugs, your good health can be prolonged for a very long time. Knowing your HIV status could save someone else's life as well as your own. Early knowledge of infection is now recognized as a critical component in controlling the spread of HIV. Once people are diagnosed, they tend to decrease behaviors that transmit HIV. Because medical treatment that lowers HIV viral load might also reduce risk for transmission to others, early medical care could prevent HIV transmission while reducing a person's risk for illness and death.

Antibody Tests

Several different tests are available to measure antibodies to HIV in blood. People choosing to have an antibody test done should be aware that it takes up to 3 months for these antibodies to develop, and in some cases up to 6 months. So if you are concerned about exposure to HIV, keep in mind that an antibody test may be negative if you are tested less than 3 months after exposure. The following tests can be used to check blood for antibodies to HIV.

An **ELISA (enzyme-linked immunosorbent assay)** is the most commonly used test to look for HIV antibodies. If antibodies are present, a confirmatory test called a Western Blot analysis is then done. Results are generally available within a few days to 2 weeks.

Oral HIV tests are now available as alternatives to blood tests. A health care provider swabbing the inside of your mouth can take a tissue sample, and the saliva is then tested for antibodies to HIV.

A **home HIV test** became available in 1997. The FDA, as a test, currently approves a test called HomeAccess for HIV. You just draw a blood sample by pricking your finger, and then you send the sample to a laboratory for antibody testing along with a personal identification number (no names are involved, so your privacy is guaranteed). A trained counselor gives you your results over the phone within several days.

Currently, the FDA has licensed one **rapid HIV test** for commercial use. The Murex Single Use Diagnostic System (SUDS) HIV Test is a manually performed, visually read, 10-minute test for the detection of antibodies to HIV. A health care provider draws a blood sample, and then the SUDS HIV Test utilizes a specialized enzyme procedure. A positive finding should be repeated to confirm it. If it is still positive, a confirmatory Western Blot test must be done, which may take several days or a week.

Tests to Determine Viral Load

Once an antibody test determines that you have been exposed to HIV, a plasma viral load test (also called a PVL test) will often be ordered to measure just how much of the HIV virus is in your blood. Your viral load will be used to customize your medications and treatment.

Three different PVL tests are commonly used: the **RT-PCR test**, the **bDNA test**, and the **NASBA test**. All of these tests work well. However, each of them can give a slightly different number for the amount of HIV in your blood, so it is wise to use the same test each time you measure your viral load.

Reliability

Standard tests, like the ELISA and Western Blot, have sensitivity and specificity rates greater than 98 percent for HIV detection.

The risk of false positives for ELISA testing for HIV is very low (0.0004 to 0.0007 percent). If you have a positive ELISA test for HIV antibodies, the first thing that will happen is that the test will be done again to confirm it. You will subsequently be tested to confirm the presence of the virus itself in your blood with an RT-PCR or similar test, further decreasing the likelihood of a false-positive finding.

False negatives are also rare and are usually due to ELISA testing prior to the production of HIV antibodies. If you are at high risk for HIV infection, especially due to a recent event (high risk sex, needlestick) and have a negative ELISA, you should retest yourself in 6 months. Alternatively, you can talk to your doctor about doing an RT-PCR or similar test to test directly for the presence of the virus now.

It is important to note that although the vast majority of people in the United States who are HIV positive are infected with the HIV-1 virus, there are some individuals who will be infected with HIV-2. Many of the ELISA screening tests are falsely negative in 20 to 30 percent of patients infected with HIV-2. If you are at high risk for HIV-2 infection (you are West African, a sexual partner of a West African, received a blood transfusion in West Africa, or were born of an HIV-2–infected mother), then you should request the specific HIV-2 test if your HIV-1 test is negative.

Health Risks

There are no medical risks for the test, as they simply require a blood draw or a saliva sample.

However, as with genetic testing (see HNPCC Genetic Tests for Cancer Risk, on page 192), there may be significant privacy and financial risks if your insurance provider or employer finds out that you have tested positive for AIDS. If you already have insurance, especially if it is a group plan through your employer, they will probably not drop your coverage if you test positive for HIV. This also usually means they will pay for your medications as well.

On the other hand, if you do not currently have insurance and find you are HIV positive, you are likely to have trouble getting insurance. You can check into the AIDS Drug Assistance Program (ADAP), a program funded by the federal government to help pay for HIV drugs. Your local ADAP office can give you more information about income requirements and which drugs it covers.

Medicaid may also be able to help you purchase HIV drugs. Medicaid is a government-sponsored insurance program that covers healthcare and medications. If you are disabled, not working, or have a low income, you may qualify for Medicaid. Like ADAP, each state has its own program, so you will need to talk to a local Medicaid worker in order to apply.

Cost of the Screening Tests

Standard tests like ELISA and Western Blot can cost anywhere from around $45 to $150.

BRCA1 AND BRCA2 GENETIC TESTS FOR BREAST AND OVARIAN CANCER RISK

As seen in the chapters on breast cancer and ovarian cancer, the presence of one or both of the BRCA1 and -2 gene mutations confers a significantly increased lifetime risk for the development of these conditions. Therefore, we recommend genetic testing for these mutations in women whose family history suggests that a BRCA gene mutation is present.

The mode of inheritance of these mutations is *autosomal dominant*, which means that only one copy of the mutated gene is required to produce the risk. For a long time, it was thought that breast cancer susceptibility was inherited only through the maternal relatives. This is not the case with the BRCA genes. Cases of breast and ovarian cancer may skip a generation when being carried by a male, but the mutation itself will occur in females in the next generation.

If You Already Have Breast Cancer

Many women who have already developed breast cancer may not see the need to be tested for BRCA mutations. There are, however, treatments that are designed specifically for BRCA-positive women that could be of great benefit. Also, you may want to help other family members to take preventive measures against breast cancer, if in fact you find a BRCA mutation is present in your family.

When it is decided through genetic counseling that genetic screening should be performed for the first member of a family, **complete sequencing of the genes** is warranted, testing the entire sequence of the BRCA genes for any mutations. This means that the entire DNA sequence of the BRCA genes will be determined and compared to the known normal sequence.

As opposed to the "shotgun" approach in full gene sequencing, families with at least one member with known BRCA1 or BRCA2 gene mutations can be tested for that specific mutation, or change. This is done by **sequencing only a small portion of the patient's DNA** where the mutation is known to exist in the relatives. If the test is negative for the known family mutation, then the individual has not inherited that specific mutation. This type of genetic testing is done to look for the three common BRCA gene mutations that are found in Ashkenazi Jewish populations.

It is important to reiterate that although having BRCA1 and -2 gene mutations puts you at significantly higher lifetime risk for breast and ovarian cancer, *it does not mean that you will definitely get these diseases*. It simply means that you are at above-average risk, but you may never get either cancer in your lifetime.

Finally, it is important to recognize that around one-third to one-half of all breast cancers that seem to run in families do not show any linkage to either BRCA1 or BRCA2 gene mutations. Again, if you have a strong family history of breast cancer and have a negative finding for BRCA gene mutations, do not become lax on medical monitoring for early detection of this cancer. There are undoubtedly other inheritable gene mutations that cause breast cancer that are simply not known at this time.

Reliability

FALSE NEGATIVE

An important aspect of genetic testing for BRCA mutations is the enormous number of mutations reported to date in these breast cancer genes. Because there are so many BRCA mutations known, sequencing of the genes is the only reliable way to screen them. However, such sequencing is time-consuming, difficult, and costly. Furthermore, not every mutation associated with breast or ovarian cancer will always be detected. The link between breast cancer and the mutation data for the families in the International Breast Cancer Consortium suggests that *up to 30 percent* of mutations escape detection.

The bottom line is this: BRCA gene sequencing is not an exact science, since there are several complexities involved in interpreting the gene sequence information, and false negatives can occur. However, if you are in fact at high risk for breast cancer based on the known risk factors, then a negative finding on BRCA testing does not mean you should let down your guard in terms of surveillance for breast cancer.

FALSE POSITIVE

BRCA genetic testing will occasionally detect changes in the BRCA gene sequence called polymorphisms (meaning "many forms"). Very often these changes do not impair the way the BRCA gene works, and hence do not increase your risk of breast or ovarian cancer—thus, detection of one of these harmless polymorphisms in the BRCA genome would be a false positive.

This is why it is important to be at high risk for breast cancer before getting tested for BRCA gene mutations—the higher your risk for getting breast cancer, the less likely the chance of having a false-positive result on BRCA testing.

Health Risks

There are no health risks in the procedure itself; for the patient, it is merely a blood draw. However, there is a privacy risk to this procedure, and that is why some people may wish to pay to have this test done—so that their insurance companies cannot find out if they are positive for one or both of these gene mutations. See HNPCC Genetic Tests for Cancer Risk, on page 192, for a more detailed look at the potential privacy risks of genetic testing.

Cost of the Tests

Tests for complete sequencing for BRCA mutations currently cost nearly $3,000. Insurance companies often cover the costs of BRCA1 and -2 genetic screening for women with more than a 10 percent chance of having this gene mutation, based on their personal and family history. But many people elect not to request reimbursement because of privacy concerns.

If a mutation is found, other members of the family only need to be tested for that specific mutation. The cost for this test is only around $350. In the Ashkenazi Jewish population, there are only three specific mutations that need to be tested for; testing each of the three also costs around $350.

Genetic counseling is free at some research centers, while other hospitals charge from $75 to $200. Insurance coverage varies.

C-REACTIVE PROTEIN TEST FOR
CORONARY HEART DISEASE RISK

C-reactive protein (CRP) is a protein secreted by the liver in response to inflammation in the body. A high concentration of CRP in the blood (i.e., an elevated CRP level) can indicate inflammation anywhere in the body, including the arteries.

Chronic inflammation in the arteries plays a major role in atherosclerosis, and thus in coronary heart disease (CHD) and carotid artery disease. CRP also appears to be more than just a marker for the presence of inflammation. Researchers have shown that CRP can actually help trigger blood clots (a major cause of heart attacks and strokes). Other researchers have shown that CRP produces direct biochemical changes in the arterial wall that can promote atherosclerosis.

Measuring Blood CRP Levels

Traditional CRP blood tests usually don't detect CRP levels below 5 mg/L, even though a result higher than 1 mg/L begins to put you at above-average risk of CHD. That's because it was believed previously that blood CRP levels below 5 mg/L were normal, and only higher levels had to be evaluated. We now know that lower levels need to be evaluated as well. Note that some labs may report blood CRP levels as milligrams per deciliter (mg/dl) instead of mg/L. If this occurs, multiply mg/dl by 10 to convert it to mg/L.

A new, high-sensitivity (HS) test for CRP has been developed that can measure serum CRP levels as low as 0.1 mg/L. Many studies have now found that CRP levels of 1 mg/L or higher begin to elevate your risk for future development of CHD or stroke, with the average risk increasing as your CRP level increases. In other words, a person with a CRP level of 5 mg/L is at greater risk of developing CHD or stroke than a person with a CRP level of 1 mg/L.

HOW DO I LOWER MY LEVEL?

Ideally, you want your blood CRP level to be below 1 mg/L. If you decide your CRP level is too high, there are a few ways to try and lower it. For starters, if you are overweight, do your best to get your weight down. If you are a smoker, quitting will not only lower your serum CRP, but provide many other health benefits as well. As noted, having a couple of drinks a day (but no more) can also significantly lower serum CRP levels. If you are a postmenopausal woman using hormone replacement therapy (HRT) and discover you have a high CRP level, you may want to discuss the benefits versus risks of estrogen replacement therapy (ERT) with your doctor.

Beyond that, two drug therapies are available. Cholesterol-lowering statin drugs and triglyceride-lowering fibrates have been found to also reduce serum CRP levels. These are potent and expensive drugs, so a decision to try them should only be made after discussing the option with a knowledgeable physician. If you find you have an elevated CRP level but you are unable to lower it, you at least are now aware that you

Therefore, measuring your blood CRP level with an HS CRP test can give you valuable information about your risk of future CHD and/or stroke.

Overnight fasting before you have your blood drawn is preferred. A few studies have shown that levels of CRP can fluctuate moderately from day to day in some people due to a wide variety of causes—like a small infection due to a paper cut or a mild viral infection. Therefore, try to have your serum CRP levels tested when you have no other concurrent health problems, like a cold or a bacterial infection, since any type of infection can temporarily elevate serum CRP levels.

need to monitor your health more vigilantly and try to minimize all of the other risk factors for CHD and CVD as aggressively as possible.

Since CRP is a marker of inflammation, finding the cause of that inflammation and controlling it—thus bringing CRP levels back down—is another approach to lowering levels. There is accumulating evidence that infection with bacteria called *C. pneumoniae* (*Chlamydia pneumoniae*) may be an important factor in the development of CHD. Therefore, people with chronically elevated CRP levels should consider being tested for antibodies to *C. pneumoniae* infection. If that infection is present, antibiotic therapy can be used to decrease the risk of developing CHD both by eradicating the infection and by lowering CRP levels once the source of the infection is removed. However, be aware that antibiotic therapy is not always successful in eradicating a chronic *C. pneumoniae* infection, so be sure to follow up with your doctor.

The best way to know your true baseline CRP level is to have it checked under fasting conditions at least twice when you feel perfectly healthy, at least a month apart, and by the same laboratory.

If you have a low blood CRP level but high cholesterol levels, you still have a higher risk of developing CHD—that has not changed. Of course, you are much better off than if your CRP were elevated, but you are by no means home free; you still need to do something about lowering your cholesterol.

Reliability

Studies supporting a link between chronic inflammation, high CRP level, and development of CHD have been accumulating over the past 10 years. Perhaps the most convincing evidence was published in the November 14, 2002 issue of *The New England Journal of Medicine*. This report was derived from the Women's Health Study, a large ongoing study evaluating ways to prevent cardiovascular events in women over 45 years of age. This component of the study tracked the health of 27,939 women for 8 years.

Elevated CRP level was actually found to be a stronger predictor of future CHD and stroke than was LDL (bad) cholesterol! Furthermore, the risk of developing CHD increased linearly as CRP levels increased from 0.49 mg/L to greater than 4.2 mg/L (remember, this is the range of blood CRP levels that doctors previously thought was normal and did not have to be evaluated). Women in this study with high CRP but low LDL cholesterol levels were at greater risk for future cardiovascular disease and stroke compared to women with low CRP levels and high LDL cholesterol. Ironically, it is only women with a poor cholesterol profile that would commonly be treated to reduce their risk of future CHD or cardiovascular disease.

The HS CRP tests have been shown to be highly sensitive and specific for measuring CRP. In the past few years, it was difficult to find laboratories that were doing the new HS CRP tests. Happily, that has changed, as we found almost all of the labs we surveyed were using the new HS CRP tests. Those who were still using the traditional tests were able to send their samples to others who could use the HS CRP tests. Bottom line: Have your doctor request the high-sensitivity test on the lab request.

Health Risks

There are none. It is a simple blood test.

Cost

The average cost of an HS-CRP test ranges from $25 to $50.

CA-125 AND TVU TESTS
FOR OVARIAN CANCER

The **carcinogenic antigen (CA) 125 blood test** measures levels of a protein that is normally confined within a cell. If, however, cell walls are inflamed or damaged, the protein may be released into the bloodstream. Ovarian cancer cells may produce an excess of these protein molecules, and therefore the CA-125 test can help in diagnosing and monitoring this disease.

It's important to remember that simply measuring blood levels of CA-125 alone *cannot* effectively find early ovarian cancer. In many early-stage ovarian cancers, this molecule is not necessarily released in large amounts. False positives can also occur, as other conditions (endometriosis, the first trimester of pregnancy, or non-gynecological cancers) will elevate CA-125. In conjunction with a **transvaginal ultrasound** (TVU) screening, however, the CA-125 test can be very effective.

A transvaginal ultrasound, also known as an endovaginal ultrasound, involves the use of sound waves to delineate internal structures with a transducer placed in the vagina.

For this test, you lie on an examining table, on your back. A light sheet is provided to cover you during the procedure. A small

THE IMPORTANCE
OF EARLY DIAGNOSIS

As with all other cancers described in this book, survival from ovarian cancer is closely related to the stage of the cancer at diagnosis. Most women with epithelial ovarian cancer, the most common form, are found to have Stage III or IV cancer by the time they develop symptoms and go to their doctors. The 5-year survival rate for these women is less than 25 percent. In contrast, the minority of patients who discover that they have early-stage ovarian cancer (cancer still confined to the ovaries) have a 5-year survival rate of 80 to 90 percent! Therefore, discovering the disease in its early, asymptomatic stages is of life-or-death importance.

handheld transducer that is covered with a latex condom is inserted into your vagina. The transducer produces images that can be seen on a video monitor, and a hard copy can be made on film. The test is completely painless and does not take much time.

Transvaginal ultrasound imaging is recommended for ovarian cancer screening in asymptomatic women at high risk for developing ovarian cancer. In a 1997 study of 14,469 women with no symptoms of ovarian cancer, researchers detected 17 ovarian cancers with TVU. Women who had abnormal findings on the first screening underwent additional tests to make sure the abnormality was not an ovarian cyst. Those who found that they did not have cysts then underwent a series of blood and ultrasound tests to determine whether there was a need for surgery. After surgery, researchers determined that 11 of the 17 cancers were Stage I (early stage). Although the total number of ovarian cancers detected was small, *65 percent* of these tumors were detected at a stage when they are most likely to be curable.

Our Recommendations

WOMEN AT HIGH RISK FOR OVARIAN CANCER

The risk table in Ovarian Cancer, on page 118, will tell you your risk level. Women at high risk for ovarian cancer should have a baseline TVU combined with a blood CA-125 measurement, followed by an annual CA-125 measurement and a TVU every 2 years. The TVU should be followed up more frequently if CA-125 is found to rise significantly from one year to the next and there are no other problems that can explain the rise.

Of these women, those with a strong family history of *either* ovarian *or* breast cancer (two or more first-degree relatives have or had the disease) should begin TVU and CA-125 screening 5 years prior to the earliest age of onset in their family.

WOMEN AT MODERATE RISK

Women in the moderate-risk category should discuss their individual circumstances with their doctor to determine the best course of action. Monitoring blood levels of CA-125 annually for significant elevations from one year to the next, beginning at age 40, is one logical option for these women.

WOMEN AT LOW RISK

Women who are at low risk for ovarian cancer should probably not be screened with TVU, as the percentage of women screened who are likely to benefit will be very small. As with moderate-risk women, an annual CA 125 test, beginning at age 40, is a good idea.

OVARIAN BIOPSY

It is important to recognize that the role of all the above tests is to simply identify a mass on the ovaries that should not be there—this is the first step in diagnosing ovarian cancer. Once women are identified as having a mass, only an accurate biopsy of the tissue can determine if it is in fact cancer.

One of the most common ways to biopsy an ovarian mass is with a CT scan-guided needle biopsy. For this procedure, the patient remains on the CT scanning table, while a radiologist advances a biopsy needle toward the location of the mass. CT scans are repeated until the doctors are confident that the needle is within the mass. A fine needle biopsy sample (tiny fragment of tissue) or a core needle biopsy sample (a thin cylinder of tissue about 1/2 inch long and less than 1/8 inch in diameter) is removed and examined for cancer cells under a microscope by a pathologist.

We cannot stress enough that early screening for ovarian cancer is underutilized by women who are at elevated risk for the disease in this country. A report in *Gynecologic Oncology* from researchers at the Fred Hutchinson Cancer Research Center in Seattle stated that "women at highest risk for ovarian cancer receive less screening and report less worry about getting the disease than women with a lower risk."

Their report revealed that while more than 60 percent of those women at elevated risk for ovarian cancer reported having undergone screening for breast cancer, less than half (47 percent) of the high-risk women said they had been screened for ovarian cancer.

"Most of the highest-risk women for ovarian cancer are at high risk because their relatives have had *breast cancer,* not ovarian cancer," the report states. "However, it appears that many of these women don't make the association between a family history of breast cancer and increased ovarian cancer risk. The connection isn't as obvious as it would be if their mother or sister, for example, had ovarian cancer."

Health Risks of the Screening Tests

There are essentially no health risks associated with either the TVU or the CA-125 blood tests.

Cost of the Tests

A TVU currently runs about $200 to $250, a CA-125 blood test about $60. Women who carry BRCA1 or -2 gene mutations may be able to get their health insurance companies to pay for these screening exams, due to their greatly increased risk. However, if you have these mutations but have not informed your insurance company, you may not want to ask for reimbursement for these tests based on your higher risk. For a more in-depth discussion of the politics surrounding genetic testing, see HNPCC Genetic Tests for Cancer Risk, on page 192.

Another possible option for women concerned about ovarian cancer is to inquire about enrolling in the Risk of Ovarian Cancer Algorithm Study (ROCA). Women who participate in the ROCA study will have their CA-125 serum levels checked every 3 months for 1 or 2 years, and a TVU of the ovaries also may be recommended. For more information, go to the Cancer Genetics Network (CGN) Web site (http://epi.grants.cancer.gov/ovarian/). Several different medical centers across the United States are participating in this study.

COLONOSCOPY
FOR COLORECTAL CANCER
AND PRECANCEROUS POLYPS

For a colonoscopy, a physician passes an endoscope up the entire length of the colon, so the procedure can find early signs of cancer in the entire colon. It also enables the physician to see inflamed tissue, other abnormal growths, ulcers, and bleeding.

For this procedure, you'll have to undergo complete bowel cleansing the evening prior to the exam. The colonoscopy is generally done in a hospital setting by a specialist (gastroenterologist). You will probably be given pain medication and a mild sedative to keep you comfortable and to help you relax during the exam.

Virtual colonoscopy is a new test for detecting polyps or colon cancer that combines a CAT (computer assisted tomography) scanner and sophisticated image processing computers with skilled radiologists to virtually recreate and evaluate the inner surface of the colon.

In this procedure, the CAT scanner provides the x-ray images, and the image processing computers create the 3-D display for the final interpretation by the radiologist. As with colonoscopy, the patient has to undergo complete bowel cleansing the evening prior to the exam. On the day of the exam, the patient lies on the CAT scan cradle. A thin tube (about the size of a rectal thermometer) is then placed in the rectum, through which air is introduced into the colon. The patient then holds his breath while the machine sweeps over the abdomen. The procedure is repeated with the patient lying on his stomach. The whole procedure takes about 10 minutes.

Although this procedure may prove to be at least somewhat more comfortable than a full colonoscopy, as of this writing it is still not proven to be as effective as a regular colonoscopy. However, patients who simply do not wish to have a colonoscopy for whatever reason should investigate this procedure as their second choice. The test is also easier for frail or elderly patients.

Overall, screening for colorectal cancer lags far behind screening for other cancers. Findings from the National Health Interview Survey (administered by the Centers for Disease Control and Prevention) indicate that in 2000, only 45 percent of men and 41 percent of women age 50 years or older had undergone a sigmoidoscopy or colonoscopy within the previous 10 years or had used a fecal occult blood test within the preceding year. Use of screening tests for colorectal cancer was particularly low among people without health insurance and people who reported no doctor's visits within the preceding year.

However, if you decide you need to be screened for colorectal cancer, colonoscopy clearly has the greatest value of currently available screening tests. Recent studies published in the *New England Journal of Medicine* have concluded that a full colonoscopy is the most effective screening tool to find colorectal cancer or precancerous polyps.

Reliability

The sensitivity of colonoscopy is very high for detection of colorectal cancers or precancerous polyps, ranging from 95 percent to

close to 100 percent in the hands of an experienced gastroenterologist. The incidence of false negatives is very low, since any suspicious lesions are biopsied during the procedure, and the subsequent
pathology workup on the tissue is the gold standard for determining whether a lesion is cancerous.

Health Risks

The risks are minimal. The two most serious complications are
bleeding and perforation of the colon, but these happen in less than
2 percent of all colonoscopies performed. Deaths related to
colonoscopy (from lower GI bleeding or from heart attack) occur
only very rarely.

Cost

A full colonoscopy can cost anywhere from $800 up to $1,500 or
more. The expense is mostly due to the fact that the procedure has
to be done in a hospital setting, so there is an additional hospital
charge for the use of the surgical suites and equipment.

If you are a Medicare recipient, however, you may be able to
have Medicare pay for 80 percent of a screening colonoscopy. Beginning July 1, 2001, Medicare expanded its coverage of colorectal
cancer screenings by funding colonoscopies for all its beneficiaries.
Medicare beneficiaries who have a history of inflammatory bowel
disease (such as ulcerative colitis or Crohn's disease) or polyps, or
who have a family history (a sibling, parent, or child with it) of colorectal cancer are eligible for more frequent screenings. Medicare
covers colonoscopies for this high-risk group every 2 years.

DEXA SCAN FOR OSTEOPOROSIS

This is the most accurate test available for diagnosing osteoporosis and risk for osteoporosis, and is generally considered
to be the gold standard of bone density measurement. It is most
often used to measure bone density of your spine and hip.

We believe that a DEXA scan of both the hip and spine is the
best method to evaluate your bone mass density (BMD). Both the
hip and spine should be scanned, because up to 25 percent of patients will have inaccurate results if only one site is evaluated. The
DEXA scan will determine whether or not you currently have osteopenia or osteoporosis, and it will predict your risk for future
fractures.

This test is easy, painless, and noninvasive. Virtually no preparation is needed on your part. If you are having the test done at a
medical center or hospital, you may not even have to change into
a gown, although you probably will be asked to remove any articles of clothing containing metal.

Interpreting Your Results

Bone density is described in relationship to what it should be in
young women. It is expressed as a "T-score," measured in standard

deviations, or SDs (statistics that compare your bone density to "normal" bone density). A committee of the World Health Organization created four diagnostic categories: normal, osteopenia, osteoporosis, and established osteoporosis.

- Normal bone density is indicated by a T-score that is less than 1 SD from the standard value.

- Osteopenia (bone density that is somewhat low) is indicated by a T-score that is between 1 and 2.5 SDs below the standard value.

- Osteoporosis is indicated by a T-score that is more than 2.5 SDs below the standard value.

- Established osteoporosis is indicated by a T-score that is more than 2.5 standard deviations below the standard value, and by the presence of fragility fractures.

Reliability

A DEXA scan is more sensitive than ordinary x-rays, more accurate than radiograms (radiographic absorptiometry), and can diagnose bone loss at a very early stage. DEXA scanning of the spine and hip have reported sensitivities for osteoporosis ranging from 70 to 90 percent, and specificities ranging from 60 to 85 percent.

Health Risks of a DEXA Scan

There is essentially no risk. During the test, you lie on a padded platform for just a few minutes while an imager—a mechanical armlike device—passes over your body. Radiation exposure is about 1/50 the amount in a standard chest x-ray.

Cost of the Screening Test

The cost of this screening test ranges between $100 and $200.

DUPLEX ULTRASOUND
FOR CAROTID ARTERY DISEASE

A number of different ultrasound tests for assessing the carotid arteries are available. One, called **B-mode imaging**, provides images of various planes of the carotid artery, allowing the computer to create a three-dimensional image of the artery wall and surrounding structures. This technique provides information on the type and extent of damage, but it cannot fully determine how blocked the carotid artery is. Therefore, B-mode imaging is often combined with another type of ultrasound called **pulsed Doppler scanning**. The pulsed Doppler test measures the speed of blood flow through an artery. Because plaque buildup narrows these arteries, the blood speeds up past the point of the plaque, so the greater the blood velocity, the narrower the blood vessel. Together, the two are known as **duplex ultrasound,** and they can provide excellent information on the status of the carotid arteries.

In this procedure, you'll be asked to lie on your back while a jellylike material is applied to your neck. Next, the technician (called a sonographer) places a small, handheld ultrasound probe over the carotid arteries.

Interpreting Your Results

It is important to remember that most asymptomatic people at risk for stroke who undergo carotid duplex ultrasound will be found to have only minimal or moderate plaque buildup in their carotid arteries. Now armed with this information, they can begin a treatment plan that involves lifestyle changes and possibly medications, so they do not advance to severe carotid artery disease.

A small percentage of asymptomatic people at risk for stroke who undergo carotid duplex ultrasound will find they already have significant carotid artery disease that requires carotid endarterectomy surgery. While a carotid endarterectomy is fairly safe surgery, it does carry certain risks, the most severe of which are stroke and death in a small percentage of patients. If your neurosurgeon recommends a carotid endarterectomy, you should be aware of these complications. More important, you should find out the complication rate for the particular surgeon and hospital performing the procedure.

Reliability

The journal *Annals of Vascular Surgery* reported in July 2002 on the value of duplex ultrasound in grading the severity of carotid artery disease. The study compared the findings of duplex ultrasound to cerebral angiography (the gold standard test for carotid artery disease) in 163 patients. In 93 percent of the patients with carotid artery disease, findings with duplex ultrasound were very similar to the findings using cerebral angiography. Furthermore, duplex ultrasound grading of the severity of the carotid artery disease was determined to be reliable and accurate.

In general, the carotid duplex ultrasound has 83 to 86 percent sensitivity and 89 to 94 percent specificity for detecting carotid artery disease in patients who have greater than 70 percent blockage of their carotid artery.

Health Risks

Carotid duplex ultrasound is essentially risk-free. Since it is a very safe procedure, there is little risk when performing it outside of the hospital or clinical setting, like in an independently run mobile medical testing unit.

Cost of the Screening Test

The cost of a carotid duplex ultrasound when performed in a clinic or hospital is between $500 and $600, including doctor's fee. This cost is much less expensive than the only slightly more sensitive and specific **magnetic resonance angiography** (MRA). Most health insurers will *not* cover the cost of this test unless your risk factors are very high—higher by far than our suggested threshold for undergoing testing for CAD.

However, we recommend having the carotid duplex ultrasound done by a private screening company, like Life Line Screening of America, where the charge is only $45 for the *exact same procedure.*

Let us say a word about these private companies that offer carotid duplex ultrasound and other tests. On the one hand, as we have noted in the introduction, some of the services they offer are unnecessary and generate far too many false positives, like the full-body CT scan. But on the other hand, for a test like the carotid duplex ultrasound, these companies offer fully competent services at a fraction of the price you would pay at a hospital (primarily because you are not paying for all the overhead costs of running the hospital).

EBCT FOR CORONARY
HEART DISEASE

As a part of the process of atherosclerotic plaque formation, calcium deposits develop in the coronary arteries along with fatty streaks. As the plaque builds up and hardens, the artery narrows and blood flow is restricted. In the worst-case scenario, the plaque ruptures or a clot forms, causing complete blockage in one or more coronary arteries—leading to a heart attack.

An electron beam computed tomogram (EBCT) is a high-tech CT scanner used to evaluate the amount of calcium in the coronary arteries of the heart. EBCT scanning produces images of your organs at 1/20 of a second—much faster than traditional CT scanners, MRI scanners, or other imaging machines. Since it takes pictures so much faster, the camera is not affected by the beating of the heart muscle and blood flow, so the resulting images are clearer and easier to read than other images.

"EBCT is the single greatest advance in the early diagnosis of heart disease," reports cardiologist Jim Grattan, M.D., EBCT Medical Director at the Covenant Medical Group in Lubbock, Texas.

An EBCT is safe, fast (10 to 15 minutes), and painless. If you are a man over 35, a woman over 45, or a woman who has had a complete ovariohysterectomy prior to age 30, and you have two or more of the common risk factors for CHD, you should get an EBCT scan. As with other tests to detect CHD, the more risk factors you have, the more likely you are to benefit from an EBCT scan.

Interpreting Your Results

The EBCT test produces a "calcium score" that indicates the extent of calcium deposits in the coronary arteries.

Normal coronary arteries are free of plaque and should have a score of zero (no calcium detected). A positive test means calcium deposits were found in the coronary arteries. This indicates at least some degree of atherosclerosis, and therefore the presence of early CHD, or the beginnings of future CHD (depending on the amount found). Since the amount of calcium found is related to the amount of atherosclerosis present, the amount detected will guide your doctor in recommending appropriate treatment (if in fact any is needed). Naturally, a higher calcium score will lead to a more aggressive treatment plan.

An EBCT scan is really a first line of defense in knowing your CHD (or potential CHD) status. However, if your EBCT scan finds a high calcium score in one or more coronary arteries, an isotope treadmill stress test may be the next step to further evaluate the possible presence of atherosclerosis (see ITST for Carotid Artery Disease and Coronary Heart Disease, on page 199).

This test is generally not recommended for patients who have irregular heartbeats, because the results are less accurate in these cases. Also, this test is generally not recommended for patients who have already had a heart attack and therefore have known heart disease.

Reliability

Studies have shown that EBCT has a higher rate of false positives than is desirable. Approximately 30 to 50 percent of the people with a high calcium score on EBCT will find out they do not have significant coronary blockage.

So, if your EBCT scan shows you have a low calcium score, you can be quite certain that you do not currently have significant atherosclerosis in your coronary arteries. But on the other hand, if you come up with a high calcium score that suggests CHD or significant coronary plaque buildup, you should undergo further testing to confirm the EBCT's findings. The follow-up test is often an ITST— an Isotope Treadmill Stress Test.

Remember, more than half of the people in whom an EBCT scan suggests early CHD find out subsequently that they *in fact do have a problem*. Therefore, this scan could very easily be the only reason these people do not become another number in heart disease and stroke statistics.

Health Risks of the EBCT

The only risk of an EBCT is some exposure to x-ray radiation. The amount of radiation is not insignificant, but it is less radiation than a traditional CT scan. You stay fully clothed, and the entire scan takes only a few minutes. There are no shots, no dyes to drink or inject, and no medications to take. It isn't even claustrophobic. You will simply lie on your back and when asked, you will hold your breath for a few seconds at a time. In fact, one of the first questions most people ask after their scan is: "Is that it?"

Cost

At this date, the cost is around $500 for a single EBCT. This may be money well spent. Many experts now believe that as more people have EBCTs, conventional tests for heart disease will be phased out, and intervention procedures such as angioplasty or bypass surgery will be greatly reduced. That's because an EBCT scan showing significant coronary artery plaque buildup will be the wake-up call that many asymptomatic people need to finally get serious about making the lifestyle changes that will prevent them from ever getting a stroke or CHD. Therefore, EBCT scans could become part of the answer to the spiraling cost of health care.

EGD FOR ESOPHAGEAL CANCER
AND STOMACH CANCER

When the physician performs an esophagogastroduodeno-scopy (EGD), she always checks from the beginning of the esophagus, then all the way down to the end of the stomach where it becomes the small intestine, even if she is only suspicious of something in the esophagus. This is why patients who are at substantial risk for both esophageal cancer *and* stomach cancer get two tests for the price of one by having an EGD done.

Prior to the EGD, you will be required to fast overnight. In preparation for the procedure, you will be given a sedative, and an analgesic and a local anesthetic will be sprayed into your mouth to suppress the need to cough or gag when the endoscope is inserted. Also, a mouth guard will be inserted to protect your teeth and the endoscope. In some cases, an IV may be inserted to administer medications during the procedure.

You will be instructed to lie on your left side. The endoscope will then be advanced through the esophagus to the stomach and duodenum, and air will be introduced to enhance viewing. The lining of these organs is examined and tissue samples can be obtained through the endoscope if necessary. When the area has been viewed, the endoscope will be removed, and you will be asked to cough to expel the extra air. Food and liquids are restricted until your cough reflex returns. The test lasts about 30 to 60 minutes.

Interpreting Your Results

ESOPHAGEAL CANCER

If you are having an EGD because you have several risk factors for esophageal cancer but do not presently have symptoms, any esophageal cancer found is much more likely to be in its earliest stages than if you had symptoms of the disease. Remember, waiting for symptoms to appear results in only *5 to 10* percent of patients with esophageal cancer being cured. For patients whose disease is found early, especially prior to the development of symptoms, the chance of a surgical cure can rise dramatically.

Barrett's esophagus occurs as a complication of chronic gastroesophageal reflux disease (GERD), primarily in white males. In fact, approximately 10 to 15 percent of individuals with chronic symptoms of GERD develop Barrett's esophagus. There are two requirements for the diagnosis of Barrett's esophagus.

1. During an EGD of the lower esophagus, an abnormal pink lining is seen as replacing the normal whitish lining of the esophagus.

2. A biopsy of this abnormal lining shows (under the microscope) the presence of intestinal type cells that are called goblet cells because of their shape. These intestinal cells should not be in the esophagus, and this is called metaplasia.

This metaplasia in the esophagus is probably a protective or adaptive response to injury to the lining of the esophagus by stomach acid, which occurs in GERD. As Henry Appelman, M.D., a pathologist, stated: "When the gut is under stress it wants to be something else."

Unfortunately, when the "something else" is intestinal metaplasia, there is a risk that it will convert to esophageal cancer in the future. The vast majority of people with Barrett's esophagus do not go on to develop esophageal cancer, but it's important to remember that identifying people with Barrett's esophagus and monitoring them over the years is the best way to prevent death from this disease.

There are methods to determine which patients with Barrett's esophagus are *most likely* to develop esophageal cancer in the future. Dysplasia is a change in the cells lining the esophagus in which the cells actually appear cancerous. However, they don't invade surrounding tissue like true cancer cells do. Esophageal dysplasia is usually categorized in a biopsy as being high, low, or indefinite grade (indefinite grade means the pathologist is unsure whether low- or high-grade dysplasia is present). When high-grade dysplasia is diagnosed, the risk of developing cancer sooner is greater than with low-grade dysplasia. In fact, esophageal cancer may already be present.

STOMACH CANCER

Remember, premalignant cell changes occur in *most if not all* stomach cancers, prior to the transformation of these cells into a full-blown cancer. The gold standard for determining if these abnormal cells are present is to take a tissue biopsy during an EGD in high-risk people, which will then be given to a pathologist to look for the abnormal cells under a special microscope. These abnormal cells are very distinct from normal cells, and it is extremely unlikely that a trained pathologist would miss abnormal cells if they are present in the tissue sample.

However, because the treatment plan can be very invasive (surgical removal of all or part of the stomach) if highly dysplastic cells are found, a finding of this type should be confirmed by a second opinion before moving forward.

Reliability

The reliability of EGD is extremely high. When cancer is actually present, it looks very different from the normal tissue. The doctor will see it and biopsy a piece of it for the pathologist to look at under the microscope for cancer cells.

Barrett's esophagus—the precursor to esophageal cancer—is more difficult to diagnose. The reliability of the EGD for finding it can vary, due to the differing levels of skill and experience of endoscopists. However, a study published in the March 2003 issue of *Gastrointestinal Endoscopy* reported a sensitivity of 75 percent and a specificity of 98 percent overall for finding abnormal lesions in the esophagus using endoscopy.

However, you will find it very unlikely that your family physician will send you for an EGD if you complain of GERD symptoms that you have had for many years. You will probably be put on medication for stomach acid secretion and told to lay off the spicy foods—which is appropriate and will certainly help the problem, but gives you no information as to whether you already have premalignant changes in your esophagus. So it's up to you to determine if an EGD is in your future (for more information about medications for GERD and EGD surveillance in Barrett's patients, see "Esophageal Cancer and Barrett's Esophagus Available Treatments," on page 228).

Health Risks of the Screening Test

EGD is safe and well-tolerated. As with any invasive procedure, however, complications can occur. These are most often due to the medications used during the procedure or are related to endoscopic therapy. The overall complication rate of EGD is less than 2 percent, and many of these complications are minor (such as inflammation of the vein through which medication is given). However, serious ones can and do occur, and almost half of them are related to the heart or lungs. Bleeding or holes in the gastrointestinal tract may also occur, especially when tumors or narrowed areas are treated or biopsied. Overall, EGD is a relatively safe procedure, with the highest risk of complications occuring in emergency situations and in seriously ill patients.

Cost

An EGD costs about $700 to $1,000 for the doctor's fee and $500 for the hospital fee. If you have one while asymptomatic, you may have to pay for it yourself. If you have medical insurance and are subsequently found to have Barrett's esophagus, future surveillance EGDs to monitor it should be paid for by your insurance company.

ELISA FOR HEPATITIS C

An enzyme-linked immunosorbent assay (ELISA) tests for the presence of antibodies to the hepatitis C virus (HCV). Since HCV is a foreign substance, your immune system will make antibodies to it within a few months of it entering the body. In most cases (but not all), if your ELISA is negative, it means that you do not have antibodies to the HCV virus and you do not need to be tested further.

If the ELISA is positive, this generally means that there are antibodies against HCV in your blood; however, it does not necessarily mean that you have HCV. It is possible that you were infected in the past and have cleared the infection. If the ELISA is positive, your doctor will probably order follow-up tests (see below) to determine if there is still virus in your blood.

Reliability

FALSE NEGATIVE

False-negative tests are rare with the ELISA, but they *can* occur in patients whose immune systems cannot produce enough antibodies, such as people on hemodialysis and people with immune disorders like HIV. A false negative can also occur if a person is tested with ELISA less than 3 to 6 months after infection, as the body may not have had enough time to develop antibodies to the virus.

FALSE POSITIVE

In very rare cases, the ELISA may give a false-positive result in people with autoimmune disorders. However, a false positive can be confirmed with follow-up testing.

Health Risks

There are no health risks involved. The tests require only that you have blood drawn to be tested for the presence of HCV antibodies.

Cost of the Screening Test

The best way to have this test performed is through a medical laboratory, after consultation with your doctor. This test costs around $70 to $100.

However, if she feels the test is not necessary, but you remain concerned about possible infection, an FDA-approved home ELISA test kit can be purchased, with instructions on how to send your sample off to the lab. This is at a cost of about $69 for one test kit, which can be ordered from the Internet. For more information, see http://www.craigmedical.com/Hepatitis_C_Test.htm or http://www.hepatitisctesting.com.

Follow-Up Tests

HCV RNA TESTS

Unlike ELISA antibody tests, HCV RNA tests directly test for the presence of HCV. There are two types of HCV RNA tests: qualitative or quantitative. Qualitative HCV RNA tests are used to determine whether or not you have HCV. If you are at high risk for having been recently exposed to HCV, your doctor might choose to perform a qualitative HCV RNA test. That's because the HCV RNA test will be positive in as little as 1 to 2 weeks after exposure, whereas an ELISA might be negative at that time (as not enough time has passed for the virus to stimulate antibody production).

Quantitative HCV RNA tests allow your doctor to determine *how much* virus is in your blood (your viral load), and this test is often used after an ELISA shows that you have in fact been exposed to the virus. A higher viral load may not necessarily be a sign of more severe or more advanced disease, but it does help measure your response to treatment. If the viral load remains the same during therapy, it suggests that another treatment should be considered.

RIBA (Recombinant Immunoblot Assay)

RIBA is another test that detects the presence of antibodies in the blood. Often a physician will order a RIBA to confirm a positive ELISA in a person who does not appear to have risk factors. Blood banks also use the RIBA to test donated blood, especially to confirm blood samples that are determined to be HCV-positive by the ELISA.

EUS AND ERCP FOR PANCREATIC DYSPLASIA OR CANCER

The combination of the ultrasound probe and an endoscope has led to the development of **endoscopic ultrasound** (EUS) scopes, or echoendoscopes. This relatively new imaging device puts an ultrasound processor on the tip of an endoscope, allowing for improved ultrasound imaging of the gastrointestinal tract and the organs adjacent to it, including the liver, pancreas, bile ducts, and lymph nodes. Because of its unique capabilities, EUS can sometimes detect abnormalities or obtain information other imaging tests cannot.

Endoscopic retrograde cholangiopancreatography (ERCP) is used primarily to diagnose and treat conditions of the gallbladder, bile ducts, liver, pancreas, and pancreatic ducts. ERCP combines the use of x-rays and an endoscope, a long, flexible, lighted tube.

For this procedure, you will lie on your left side on an examining table and be given medication to numb your throat (to prevent gagging) and a sedative to help you relax during the exam. You will swallow the endoscope, and the physician will then guide the scope through your esophagus, stomach, and duodenum (first part of the small intestine) until it reaches the spot where the ducts of the gall bladder and pancreas open into the duodenum. You will then be turned to lie flat on your stomach, and the physician will pass a small plastic tube through his endoscope. The doctor will inject a dye through the tube into the ducts, and a radiographer will begin taking x-rays as soon as the dye is injected. If anything suspicious is seen, the doctor can take a biopsy. ERCP takes anywhere from 30 minutes to 2 hours, depending on what is found.

Reliability

The ERCP is the gold standard for diagnosing pancreatic cancer, and can detect abnormalities of the pancreas about 90 percent of the time they are present. However, a 1999 study published in the *Annals of Internal Medicine* found that using EUS as an initial screening test for pancreatic dysplasia (followed by an ERCP if pancreatic abnormalities were found) could be lifesaving tools in screening families with a family history of pancreatic cancer.

In this study, Teresa Brentnall, M.D., an Assistant Professor at the University of Washington Medical Center in Seattle, and her colleagues studied 14 patients from three large families who had two or more members in at least two generations diagnosed with pancreatic cancer.

In 10 of the 14 patients, an EUS showed suspicious changes in the pancreas. These 10 patients then had an ERCP, which showed that seven of these 10 patients had pancreatic irregularities as well. These seven patients subsequently had their entire pancreas removed, and it was found that all seven had widespread pancreatic dysplasia.

None of the 14 patients—seven who had surgery and seven who did not—has developed pancreatic cancer in the 1 to 4 years they have been followed to date. However, because EUS and ERCP are invasive and somewhat expensive procedures that carry some risk (particularly ERCP), these tests should only be sought by people who are at high risk for developing pancreatic cancer.

Health Risks

The complication rates associated with EUS are very low (about 0.05 percent). There is about a 1 in 2,000 chance of a significant complication. For patients who have some tissue taken for biopsy during their EUS, complications still only occur between 0.5 to 1 percent of the time.

The main complications of ERCP are pancreatitis, infection, and bleeding. Overall, fewer than 1 in 10 individuals will have such a complication, and severe life-threatening complications are even more rare (1 to 2 percent). Usually, ERCP can be done as a same-day procedure without the need for an overnight hospital stay.

Cost

An EUS costs about $500 for the doctor's fee and $500 for the hospital's fee. An ERCP is more expensive, usually costing between $1,500 and $2,000.

H. PYLORI TESTS
FOR STOMACH CANCER RISK

In the **urea breath test,** you swallow a capsule or drink water containing urea (a nitrogen waste product) that is tagged with carbon-13 or carbon-14. If *H. pylori* bacteria are present in your stomach, they will break down the urea, causing you to breathe out carbon dioxide containing the tagged carbon. If no *H. pylori* bacteria are present, the urea does not break down but passes out of your body in your urine.

The **blood antibody test** is a blood test done to see whether your body has made antibodies to *H. pylori* bacteria. If such antibodies are present, it means you either are infected or have been infected in the past (usually within the past 2 years). Blood tests may not always provide reliable results for people who have had a previous *H. pylori* infection. They cannot be used to determine if antibiotic treatment has eradicated *H. pylori*, because antibodies can take up to 2 years to disappear from the blood after the infection is cured.

A **stool antigen test** detects the immune substances (antigens) that trigger the immune system to fight an *H. pylori* infection. In an *H. pylori* infection, these antigens are shed in a person's feces (stool). Stool antigen testing is less expensive than the other tests, is noninvasive, and its results can be obtained quickly (in about 3 hours).

HNPCC GENETIC TESTS
FOR CANCER RISK

If your family meets the Amsterdam II criteria for HNPCC, and you or a family member have already been diagnosed with colorectal or other HNPCC-associated cancer (colorectal cancer, cancer of the endometrium, small bowel, ureter, or kidney, you should ask your surgeon about having the DNA of the cells from a tumor tested for microsatellite instability (MSI), which can point to mutations in the mismatch repair genes (MMR). **Microsatellite instability testing** is a good front line test for people with colorectal cancer who suspect that they might have HNPCC, as it is relatively inexpensive.

Approximately 95 percent of tumors from individuals with HNPCC exhibit MSI. Screening tumor specimens for MSI is often performed prior to proceeding with the more expensive **gene mutation analysis test** (see below). If a tumor is found to have MSI, you are at high risk for having an MMR gene mutation, and thus HNPCC.

At least 5 percent of tumors from people who in fact have HNPCC will be MSI *negative* (resulting in a false negative), and approximately 15 percent of tumors from people who in fact do *not* have HNPCC will exhibit MSI (resulting in a false positive).

Nevertheless, if your tumor is found to contain MSI, you should then proceed to actual genetic testing for MMR gene mutations—the gene mutation analysis test. If a particular gene mutation is found, the search for that specific mutation in other family members can be accomplished rapidly, accurately, and fairly inexpensively.

Although there are five MMR gene mutations that are known to produce HNPCC, mutations in two of these genes are thought to account for approximately 60 to 70 percent of all HNPCC cases. These genes, called hMSH2 and hMLH1, are the genes that most labs currently test for mutations.

If you yourself have never had cancer of any kind, but your family meets the Amsterdam II (or similar) criteria for HNPCC, you should discuss the possibility of having genetic testing done on a blood sample to screen for hMSH2 and hMLH1 gene mutations. Remember, prior to genetic testing of your DNA, you must undergo genetic counseling to understand what the results can and cannot tell you.

Health Risks of the Screening Test

Testing for MSI in a tumor specimen or for hMSH2 and hMLH1 gene mutations in a blood sample entails no health risks itself. However, having these tests done can trigger a *privacy and financial risk*, and that comes about if you ask your insurer to pay for these tests.

There are no cases we are aware of where HNPCC test results have been used as a basis for raising premiums or denying insurance policies for people with group health insurance plans. The Health Insurance Portability and Accountability Act (HIPPA) is intended to guarantee health insurance coverage regardless of health status and pre-existing conditions. However, this legislation does *not* provide privacy protection and does not prevent group health insurance plans from increasing group rates because of an individual's increased risk of disease. It also does not protect people insured under individual insurance plans from being denied insurance or from paying higher premiums because of pre-existing conditions.

Patients are not the only ones who have reason to be concerned about the privacy of their genetic information. The fear of genetic discrimination also creates a problem for the clinician with respect to issues of confidentiality. The medical geneticist, Dr. Kenneth Offit, writes, "Clinicians are left to choose between two bad alternatives: recording genetic data in patient charts (posing insurance risks to patients), or keeping genetic data in separate records (compromising availability of information to be used in making medical decisions)."

When testing is performed in a research setting, providers may

DOES DOCTOR KNOW BEST?

It would be unwise to just assume that your doctor knows about genetic testing for HNPCC and who would be a good candidate for genetic testing. The following was published in the *American Journal of Gastroenterology* in March 2002.

Gastroenterologists practicing in New York State were surveyed to assess their awareness of cancer genetic counseling and genetic testing for familial adenomatous polyposis (FAP) and HNPCC.

Of the 35 percent who responded, only 34 percent of these doctors were aware of the availability of genetic tests for HNPCC. Furthermore, 95 percent were aware of the issue of genetic counseling prior to having genetic tests, but only 51 percent said they would routinely refer patients for genetic

be able to obtain a certificate of confidentiality issued by the Department of Health and Human Services. The certificate protects the researcher from being compelled to reveal the identity of research subjects "in any federal, state or local civil, criminal, administrative, legislative, or other proceedings." This too, is problematic, as a clear distinction between "research" and "clinical" is often difficult to make. Certificates of confidentiality are not appropriate or available in all situations that involve genetic testing. An even greater problem may confront patients who have been tested, as they may be put in the position of having to withhold information about genetic test results if asked by an insurance company.

In short, this is why some people may wish to pay to have this test done themselves—so that their insurance companies cannot find out if they are positive for genetic disorders.

---

counseling before sending them for genetic testing. Presented with a family history consistent with HNPCC, 79 percent could identify the syndrome, but only 26 percent recommended genetic testing. A mere 16 percent advised the appropriate follow-up screening for known HNPCC patients, according to current recommendations.

As you can see, you cannot necessarily depend on your doctor's knowledge in this case. This is one area in particular where you need to be informed. We believe that those families who are at high risk for having an HNPCC gene mutation should know about and take advantage of appropriate genetic testing. There is a significant possibility that it will save their lives and the lives of their children in generations to come.

The Risk of a False Result

The sensitivity of HNPCC gene testing is limited from the start by the fact that it tests for only two of five known mismatch repair genes (hMSH2 and hMLH1). The large majority of HNPCC-related mutations occur on these two genes (126 of the 129 known mutations). It is possible for you to have one of the three mutations that do not occur on these genes, leading to a negative test result, when in fact you would be harboring such a mutation.

The risk of false positives and false negatives is an issue that patients should discuss with their genetic counselor if they choose to have these tests done. Because the sensitivity and specificity of genetic tests are not 100 percent, a negative finding in someone with a family history strongly indicative of HNPCC should be investigated further.

False negatives are also possible in MSI testing. The sensitivity of MSI testing in tumor tissue is high, but it is not 100 percent (as noted above, at least 5 percent of tumors from people who in fact have HNPCC will be MSI *negative*). Therefore, genetic testing for gene mutations should not necessarily be abandoned in patients with a negative tumor test for MSI but whose family histories are strongly indicative of HNPCC.

Cost

Charges range from $200 to $300 for MSI testing and up to $2,000 for sequence analysis for MMR gene mutations. The cost will be significantly less if you are looking for a known MMR gene mutation that has already been sequenced in another family member.

No laboratory should perform analysis for MMR gene mutations unless you have met with a genetic counselor and your family history has been evaluated and possible outcomes discussed. Make sure you do this prior to genetic testing.

HOMOCYSTEINE TEST
FOR CORONARY HEART DISEASE

Homocysteine is a natural amino acid that was first discovered in 1932. Our cells are constantly making and breaking down amino acids, and homocysteine is an intermediate compound that is formed in cells during the process of converting one type of amino acid into another.

An elevated level of homocysteine (hyperhomocysteinemia) has been identified as an independent risk factor for developing plaque buildup in the major arteries of the heart and brain (atherosclerosis) and subsequent CHD and other vascular diseases.

Recent research has found that 15 to 30 percent of patients who show signs of early atherosclerosis have a moderately elevated homocysteine, and that up to 10 percent of all cases of CHD may be due to elevated homocysteine levels. In general, the higher the homocysteine level, the higher the risk of developing atherosclerosis and CHD.

To be sure, an elevated plasma level of homocysteine is only one of several risk factors for atherosclerosis, but today it may be the least understood (even by your doctor) and most undertested risk factor for this deadly disorder.

The test for hyperhomocysteinemia is actually a simple test known by a complicated name: a *fasting blood draw for assay of total plasma homocysteine concentration*. So what does this mean?

This test is a blood test, so you'll have blood drawn. A laboratory then checks the total homocysteine level. A fasting total homocysteine level less than or equal to 12 µmol/L (micromoles of homocysteine per liter) is considered to be normal by most labs. However, levels below 10 µmol/L are desirable, because levels near the upper limit of normal are still associated with an increased risk of CHD.

There is also a genetic test to find out if you have one of the principal genetic mutations that can predispose you to getting hyperhomocysteinemia. Most centers that perform genetic testing for the most common mutations recommend that you be tested only if you already suffered a heart attack or stroke at an early age associated with a high plasma homocysteine level, or if you have a first-degree family member who has the mutation *and* an elevated homocysteine level.

Reliability

The specificity of the blood test is high. Sensitivity ranges from lab to lab, but most labs can accurately distinguish plasma homocysteine levels in the blood, in the range that is predictive of future CHD.

Health Risks of the Test

There are none. It is a simple blood draw.

Cost

The typical charge for measuring fasting plasma homocysteine ranges from $50 to $85.

ITST FOR CAROTID ARTERY DISEASE AND CORONARY HEART DISEASE

An isotope treadmill stress test (ITST) is also known as a nuclear, thallium, Cardiolite, Myoview or dual isotope stress test, depending upon which method is used. The preparation for the test and the treadmill procedure is similar to that for a regular treadmill stress test. In both, the patient is brought to the exercise laboratory where the heart rate and blood pressure are recorded at rest. Electrodes are then attached to the chest, shoulders, and hips and connected to the EKG machine. The treadmill is then started slowly, at warm-up speed. The slope and speed of the treadmill are increased every 3 minutes. Each 3-minute interval is known as a stage (stage 1, stage 2, stage 3, etc.). The patient's blood pressure is usually recorded during the second minute of each stage.

During the test, the physician pays attention to heart rate, blood pressure, changes in the EKG pattern, irregular heart rhythm, and the patient's appearance and symptoms. The treadmill is usually stopped when the patient achieves a target heart rate. However, if the patient is doing extremely well at peak exercise, the treadmill test can be continued further. The test may be stopped early if the patient develops significant chest pain, shortness of breath, or dizziness.

During exercise, healthy coronary arteries dilate more than diseased or blocked coronary arteries. The difference in dilation causes more blood to be delivered to the part of the heart muscle supplied by the normal coronary artery. In contrast, narrowed coronary arteries supply reduced flow to their area of distribution in the heart muscle.

When a nuclear isotope is injected, it travels to the heart muscle with blood flow. It is then extracted by the heart muscle in proportion to the flow of blood to the muscle. In other words, areas of the heart that have adequate blood flow quickly pick up the isotope, and heart muscle with reduced blood flow picks up the isotope slowly or not at all.

After injection of the isotope, images of the heart are taken by a special scanning camera, and this then helps identify the location, severity, and extent of reduced blood flow to the heart.

The ITST is divided into three parts: imaging at rest, a treadmill stress test, and imaging after exercise. There are two common types of isotope used in the United States: thallium and technetium. Some laboratories use a dual-isotope technique, where thallium is used for the resting images and technetium is used for the stress pictures. Depending upon the isotope and protocol for the laboratory, resting images may be obtained either before the stress test or 2 to 4 hours after.

We recommend this test for all men over 45 years of age and women over 55 years of age (or younger, if they have had a complete ovariohysterectomy prior to age 30) with *three or more* of the modifiable or nonmodifiable risk factors for CHD and CAD listed in Part Two.

Furthermore, this test should be considered by all men over 45 years of age and women over 55 years of age (or younger, if they have had a complete ovariohysterectomy prior to age 30) who are sedentary, have *two or more* risk factors for CHD and CAD, but who are planning to start a vigorous aerobic exercise program.

Reliability

The ITST is an effective way to determine if blockage is *already* present in the coronary arteries. An ITST is not a good test to find very early CHD, and this is one of the ways it differs from an EBCT test (see page 177). An abnormal finding with the ITST implies that you probably already have a greater than 50 percent blockage in one or more coronary arteries. This may result in you getting further testing (possibly a coronary angiogram, the gold standard for diagnosing coronary artery disease) to determine the actual extent of the blockage, and what, if anything, needs to be done.

If you are able to achieve the target heart rate and good quality images are obtained, an ITST has a sensitivity and specificity of around 65 percent and 85 percent, respectively. Therefore, approximately 15 percent of patients may have a false-positive test (when the result is abnormal in a patient who in fact does not have CHD). Therefore, some individuals may end up getting a coronary angiogram that is unnecessary (which will confirm that CHD is absent). People with several risk factors for CHD who are considering this test need to understand this and weigh it against the fact that an ITST *will* find CHD around 85 percent of the time when it is actually present.

It is also important to recognize that even if significant blockage of the coronary arteries is absent, you are not totally free of risk for a heart attack. Some studies indicate that even low-grade coronary artery blockage can be the source of spontaneous thrombosis—a condition where a blood clot or piece of plaque plugs the coronary artery, leading to a heart attack and sudden death. So keep taking your daily baby aspirin!

Health Risks

An ITST is extremely safe and carries with it a small potential risk of complications, probably 1 in 1,500 to 1 in 2,000 cases. These complications mainly involve rare skin rashes (usually from an allergic reaction to the isotope infusion) and generally nothing other than that. The total dose of radiation is less than that of a chest x-ray.

The following people should *not* take the ITST test.

- Asymptomatic men or women under 60 years of age who have essentially none of the major risk factors for CHD. Because CHD is uncommon in these people, there will be many more false positives, causing undue anxiety and needless, expensive follow-up testing.
- People with known CHD
- People who have certain types of arrhythmias (problems with the electrical system of the heart): ITST results are less accurate in these cases.
- Patients who have known heart problems other than CHD, such as mitral valve prolapse, aortic stenosis, cardiac inflammation, or Wolff-Parkinson-White syndrome
- People with acid-base disorders or thyroid abnormalities
- Patients who are obese: These people are less likely to get accurate results.

Cost of the Screening Test

The typical charge for an ITST ranges from $1,000 to $1,500.

LOW-DOSE SPIRAL CT SCAN
FOR LUNG CANCER

There is now renewed hope for early detection of lung cancer. The Early Lung Cancer Action Project (ELCAP) began in 1992 and has demonstrated that screening of high-risk people by low-dose spiral CT scan (LDSCT) can detect lung cancer at earlier and more curable stages than ordinary chest x-ray. The sensitivity of LDSCT is significantly superior even to that of conventional CT scanning.

The spiral CT scan is a painless procedure in which a special imaging machine rotates rapidly around the body, taking over one hundred pictures in sequence. The scan is sensitive enough to detect lung nodules that cannot be seen on a conventional x-ray.

Reliability

Claudia Henschke, M.D., Chief of the Chest Imaging Division at New York Weill Cornell Medical Center, in 1999 published one of the first studies looking at the feasibility of using LDSCT to detect early lung cancers. It was also reported on the front page of *The New York Times*. In this ELCAP study, smokers and ex-smokers,

60 and over, with no prior cancers, were screened with both an LDSCT of the chest and a conventional chest x-ray. The results showed that conventional chest x-rays *failed* to reveal 85 percent of the early-stage cancers detected by LDSCT. Of the cancers detected by LDSCT, 96 percent of these small lesions could be surgically removed.

Other studies, including a follow-up study by Dr. Henschke and her colleagues, have also suggested that LDSCT is a promising method for screening early lung cancer.

Health Risks of the Screening Test

The only risk involved is radiation exposure. However, if you are a long-time smoker, the potential benefits will far outweigh the low risks of the radiation you receive.

Availability

As of this writing, the National Cancer Institute and FDA does not accept LDSCT scanning as being a cost-effective screening tool for early detection of lung cancer. However, with the recent reported findings by ELCAP, early lung cancer screening as standard practice for persons at high risk of lung cancer could receive FDA approval in the very near future.

Because advanced lung cancer has such a poor prognosis, many hospitals are not waiting for formal approval of the FDA, but are already offering these scans to smokers, either as part of an ongoing research project or as a pay-as-you-go service.

One site where you can receive an LDSCT scan is the Weill Cornell Medical Center in Manhattan, which offers two different lung cancer screening programs. One is a research program, which offers a free screening LDSCT for individuals over 60 years of age who meet certain qualifying factors. The second is a clinical pro-

THE RISKS OF ACTING UPON
A FALSE POSITIVE

These risks need thorough consideration. As any radiologist will tell you, many of us have nodules or lesions in our lungs that are perfectly harmless and need no treatment. Because of the high sensitivity of LDSCT, many people will be found to have one or more lung nodules after this procedure, but the vast majority of these nodules will be harmless. Characteristics of the nodule may point toward it being benign (size, calcification, borders, and other indicators), but there can be no guarantee without biopsy.

People who are inveterate worriers need to consider this before they decide to undergo an LDSCT. If a small lesion is found that the radiologist believes is most likely benign, the appropriate follow-up might be to have another scan in several months or a year. Any significant interval change in size would suggest that it is likely to be malignant, and at that point further testing (biopsy) or treatment would be considered. On the other hand, if the lesion does not change over 2 years, you can be assured it is not lung cancer. If you are a worrier and cannot handle this "watchful waiting," you may demand a biopsy and end up having surgery just to put your mind at rest.

gram that benefits those who do not qualify for the research program but are still interested in having an LDSCT scan.

If you are 60 years of age or over and are interested in enrolling in the research program, you can call toll-free (866) 693-5227 or (866) NY-ELCAP for a site closest to you. Or you can call Weill Cornell Medical Center directly at (212) 746-1325 to see if you qualify and to schedule an appointment. If you do not qualify for the research program and would still like to have an LDSCT, you can enroll in the clinical program.

To schedule a clinical program appointment, you do need a prescription from your physician. Currently, most insurance plans do not cover this procedure, and a fee of approximately $300 is taken at the time of the appointment.

Another option is The International Early Lung Cancer Action Project (I-ELCAP). The I-ELCAP protocol is an updated version of the original ELCAP that began in 1992 and is updated annually based on evolving technology and research. It represents many hospitals throughout the United States and around the world that offer LDSCT scans for early lung cancer detection. However, each of these participating institutions has different guidelines, costs, and patient qualifications. To check for the nearest participating facility in your area, visit the I-ELCAP Web site, which lists participating institutions and their contact numbers: http://www.ielcap.org.

Cost of the Screening Test

Currently, the LDSCT cost runs between $300 and $500.

NMP22 TEST FOR BLADDER CANCER

This is a very new test for bladder cancer. It is a painless, non-invasive test performed on a single urine sample that measures the level of NMP22, a nuclear matrix protein (NMP). NMPs are found in the nuclei of cells, where they contribute to various cell functions. NMP22 is found in both normal and cancerous bladder cells, and these cells all release some NMP22 into the urine. Healthy individuals generally have very small amounts of this protein in their urine, but patients with bladder cancer often have elevated levels, even at the earliest stages of the disease (when they have no symptoms yet).

Clinical studies by urologists have shown the NMP22 test to be twice as sensitive as conventional urine cytology in detecting low-grade bladder cancer tumors. In a study published in the *Journal of Urology*, 608 patients were evaluated for the presence of bladder cancer using various tests. Of those patients, 52 were ultimately diagnosed with bladder cancer. Of the 52 tumors, NMP22 detected 46, for a sensitivity of 88.5 percent. There were, however, 89 false positives in the whole group.

When the authors of this study looked more closely at the false positives, they found that there were a few main reasons for the increased levels of urinary NMP22—benign inflammatory

WHAT IF I HAVE A FALSE-POSITIVE RESULT?

The false-positive rate is not insignificant for this test. Fortunately, it is a relatively simple process to rule it out. That's because a positive NMP22 would be followed by further tests, including cytoscopy, to confirm the presence of bladder cancer. Cytoscopy remains the gold standard for diagnosing bladder cancer. Although it is an invasive procedure, the risks associated with it are very low. Thus, the risk that you could go on to have unnecessary surgery or other treatment for bladder cancer based on an NMP22 test alone is almost nonexistent.

conditions, bladder stones, foreign bodies in the bladder, or presence of a different type of cancer. Therefore, by excluding these clinical categories, the specificity and sensitivity of the test increased to over 90 percent.

Health Risks of the NMP22 Screening Test

There are none. All you do is provide a urine sample.

Cost of the Screening Test

The NMP22 Test Kit is in the process of being incorporated by laboratories at many of the nation's leading medical institutions. In addition, most of the major national reference laboratories, including Laboratory Corporation of America, SmithKline Beecham Clinical Laboratories, PATH Lab, and Quest now offer the test. It costs approximately $110.

PSA TESTS FOR PROSTATE CANCER

Prostate specific antigen (PSA) was discovered in 1979. It is a protein produced by the cells that line the inside of the prostate. Prostate cancer changes the cellular barriers that normally keep PSA within the ductal system of the prostate, causing PSA to be released into the blood in higher quantities. All of the tests below consist of a simple blood draw and a laboratory analysis.

The **total PSA test** measures the total amount of PSA in your blood. The results are given in ng/ml (nanograms of PSA per milliliter blood), and a total PSA of 4 ng/ml or higher is considered to be a possible sign of prostate cancer. The risk increases as this number goes higher.

The total PSA and DRE (digital rectal examination) are generally the first line of tests done for detecting prostate cancer. If a suspicious finding occurs in either of these tests, your doctor will probably order follow-up tests, like a percent-free PSA test or transrectal prostate ultrasound, to determine if you should have a prostate biopsy.

The **PSA velocity test** is a measurement of the total PSA level over a period of time. Total PSA velocity should be determined over 24 months by measuring the total PSA on at least three separate occasions, spaced as equally apart as possible—ideally, every 8 months. A rise in total PSA of over 0.75 ng/ml per year over this time is suggestive of prostate cancer and may warrant having a prostate biopsy.

The total PSA that is measured in the blood exists in two major forms—PSA that circulates bound to proteins (the more abundant form) and PSA that circulates "free" in the blood (not bound to proteins). The **percent-free PSA test,** by measuring *only* that amount of the total PSA that is in the free form, enhances the overall reliability of the PSA test, because men with prostate cancer tend to have a lower percentage of PSA in the free form than men without prostate cancer.

The percent-free PSA test is mainly used as a follow-up test in men who are found to have a total PSA level in the so-called "gray area"—between 4 ng/ml and 9.9 ng/ml—to help determine who should undergo a prostate biopsy and who should not. Currently, a prostate biopsy is recommended in these men when their percent-free PSA is less than 10 percent. A biopsy is usually *not* recommended when their percent-free PSA is greater than 25 percent. If the percent-free PSA is between 10 and 25 percent, the patient's overall risk profile is used to decide how to proceed.

Follow-Up Testing

Once your doctor determines that you have an abnormal digital rectal examination or an abnormal PSA (based on total levels, percent-free PSA, PSA velocity, or a combination), the next step will most likely be a transrectal ultrasound of your prostate.

For the **transrectal prostate ultrasound** (TPU), a cylinder-shaped ultrasound probe will be gently placed in your rectum as you lie on your left side with your knees bent. The probe is rocked back and forth to obtain images of the entire prostate. The procedure takes about 15 to 25 minutes to perform.

The TPU can display both the smooth-surfaced outer shell of the prostate and the core tissues surrounding the urethra (the tube that comes out of the bladder down through the penis). The doctor will look at the entire volume of your prostate.

If the TPU shows an enlarged prostate, this indicates either inflammation of the prostate (prostatitis) or benign enlargement of the gland. A TPU showing either a distinct lump or an irregular area within the gland suggests cancer. If a lump or irregularity is seen, a biopsy will be taken in order to definitively diagnose cancer.

Reliability

Total PSA Test

The total level of PSA in serum is increased by factors other than cancer. So, like the DRE, total blood PSA alone is neither accurate nor optimally specific for prostate cancer screening. Only 15 to 25 percent of men with an elevated total PSA (greater than 4 ng/dL) are found to actually have prostate cancer. Similarly, up to 30 percent of men who do in fact have prostate cancer have a normal total PSA blood level.

PSA Velocity Test

This test has a reported sensitivity of about 72 percent and a specificity of 95 percent. Remember, sensitivity is the ability to detect the disease when it's truly there. Specificity is the ability to detect the absence of disease when it is truly absent. Therefore, this test is pretty good at detecting prostate cancer when you in fact have it, and it is very good at informing you that you do not have it. However, since this test is done over a 2-year period, it isn't appropriate when a quick diagnosis is necessary.

Health Risks

There are none for the various PSA tests; these are simple needle draws. And there are no serious risks from a TPU without a biopsy. Infection is rare, only occurring as a result of biopsy (if one is done) rather than as a result of the ultrasound itself.

Cost of the Screening Tests

The standard PSA blood test costs between $20 and $60. Some self-testing home kits are available for about $40 from Web sites like TestCountry.com. The free PSA blood test and the PSA velocity test cost about $100 each. Medicare and most health insurers typically cover these tests for men over 50.

THE
TREATMENTS

ABDOMINAL AORTIC ANEURYSM (AAA) TREATMENT

Small aneurysms that are dilated less than 2 inches (about 5 centimeters) rarely rupture and pose little risk to the patient. Therefore, in patients who are tested and found to have a small AAA, a "watchful waiting" plan should be developed in which the AAA is checked annually with ultrasound.

If the aneurysm is large, the risk of rupture and life-threatening bleeding increases. In most cases, physicians recommend surgical intervention of aneurysms that are dilated 5 centimeters or greater.

Surgical Management of AAA

There are two types of surgery that are currently used to repair an AAA: **abdominal surgery** and a newer procedure called **endovascular surgery**.

In traditional open abdominal surgery for repair of an AAA, the surgeon opens the abdomen, secures the aneurysm, and replaces it with a polyester cloth graft. Preparation for this surgery involves a general anesthetic and a small tube placed in your back (epidural) to help with pain relief following surgery. While you are asleep, tubes will also be inserted into your bladder to drain your urine, into your stomach (via your nose) to stop you from feeling sick, and into a vein in your neck for blood pressure measurements and administration of fluid following surgery. You will have a cut down or across your abdomen, and occasionally it is necessary to make a smaller cut in one or both sides of your groin. The aorta and the swollen area are then replaced by an artificial blood vessel. The hospital stay is usually less than 10 days, and recovery is usually complete in 4 to 6 weeks.

Not all patients are good candidates for abdominal surgery, however. Luckily, endovascular abdominal aortic aneurysm repair is available for patients who cannot have abdominal surgery. In this procedure, a stent graft is inserted into the aneurysm. The stent graft is housed inside a catheter that is inserted into the diseased vessel through a tiny incision in the groin. The catheter is then advanced to the level of the aneurysm. Once the graft is properly placed, the surgeon withdraws the catheter and the stent graft expands to fit inside the aneurysm.

You will not have to be put completely to sleep for this procedure. You will be given medication to numb the area where the incisions will be made. (You will have two small incisions, one in each side of your groin.) You will also be given medication in your IV that will make you drowsy. The amount of time required to do an endovascular abdominal aortic repair varies with each patient but on average takes 2 to 4 hours. Normally patients who have had this surgery go home in 1 to 2 days.

Endovascular abdominal aortic aneurysm repair is a relatively new procedure offered not only to healthy patients, but also to elderly or ailing patients who, because of other health issues, could not have their aneurysms repaired by the conventional procedure. Prior to this recent development, these patients did not have the option of aneurysm repair.

BLADDER CANCER TREATMENTS

Bladder cancer, like all cancers, has a much better prognosis when found before it has invaded the surrounding tissue. The sooner you are diagnosed, the greater your chances that the cancer is in its earliest stages and most amenable to treatment or even cure.

After bladder cancer is confirmed, the urologist will determine the best way to proceed. Surgery is the most common treatment for bladder cancer. The type of surgery depends largely on the stage and grade of the tumor.

Radical cystectomy: For invasive bladder cancer, the most common type of surgery is radical cystectomy. Radical cystectomy is the removal of the entire bladder, the nearby lymph nodes, part of the urethra, and nearby organs that may contain cancer cells.

Segmental cystectomy: In some cases, the doctor may remove only part of the bladder in a procedure called segmental cystectomy. This type of surgery is used if the cancer is low-grade and has invaded the bladder wall in only one area.

Transurethral resection: The doctor may treat early (superficial) bladder cancer with transurethral resection (TUR). During TUR, the doctor inserts a cystoscope into the bladder through the urethra. The doctor then uses a tool with a small wire loop on the end to remove the cancer and to burn away any remaining cancer cells.

External radiation therapy: In external radiation therapy, a large machine outside the body aims radiation at the tumor area. Most people receiving external radiation are treated 5 days a week for 5 to 7 weeks as an outpatient.

Internal radiation therapy: In this procedure, the doctor places a small container of a radioactive substance into the bladder through the urethra or through an incision in the abdomen. The radiation then kills the cancer cells and the implant is removed, leaving no radiation in the patient's body.

Intravesical chemotherapy: Intravesical chemotherapy refers to chemical treatments that are introduced into the bladder through the urethra using a catheter (a small, thin tube). These procedures are usually done in the office and require only 5 minutes to perform. The tube is removed immediately, but the medications must be kept in the bladder for about 2 hours. Because this therapy is limited to the bladder, the side effects are increased urination frequency, urgency, and burning with urination.

BREAST AND OVARIAN CANCER PREVENTION IN WOMEN WITH KNOWN BRCA GENE MUTATIONS

Below, we've included steps that can be taken to help prevent breast and ovarian cancer—even if you are at increased risk—if you discover that you have BRCA gene mutations.

Breast Cancer

Increased vigilance with very frequent monitoring: The most frequently used option for those who discover they have a genetic predisposition to breast cancer is to become extremely vigilant about detecting the early development of breast cancer. In particular, this means frequent screening mammograms. Mammograms do come with some radiation risk, but women with a high risk of developing breast cancer will probably want to begin screening considerably earlier than the usual age of 50 and repeat it as frequently as their gynecologists deem worthwhile. Women who have a breast tumor detected in its earliest stages have a much higher survival rate than women whose breast cancers are detected in more advanced stages.

Chemoprevention: Chemoprevention, the use of drugs, chemicals, or both to prevent the onset of breast cancer, is now an option for women at increased risk of developing breast cancer.

Tamoxifen is a drug that is classified as a selective estrogen receptor modulator (SERM). SERMs act like estrogen in some tissues, but block the effects of estrogen in other tissue. Tamoxifen mimics estrogen in bone, cardiovascular, and uterine tissue, but blocks estrogen in breast and ovarian tissue. It has been used for over 20 years to treat women who already have been diagnosed with estrogen-sensitive breast cancer.

Tamoxifen has now been approved by the FDA to *prevent* breast cancer in women deemed to be at high risk for the disease. The Breast Cancer Prevention Trial (BCPT) found a 49 percent decrease in invasive breast cancer in high-risk women who took tamoxifen therapy. The study showed that women taking tamoxifen also had fewer diagnoses of noninvasive breast cancer. However, this study also found that tamoxifen increased the risk of other serious problems such as pulmonary embolism, uterine cancer, deep vein thrombosis, and stroke. Women considering tamoxifen as a breast cancer preventative need to discuss the potential risks versus benefits of this drug with their doctors.

Raloxifene is another drug being studied for use in the chemoprevention of breast cancer. It is also a SERM, and has estrogen effects very similar to tamoxifen's. Unlike tamoxifen, raloxifene does not increase the risk of uterine cancer. Although a promising compound, raloxifene is not approved by the FDA as a chemopreventative drug for breast cancer as of this writing. However, it may be soon.

In 1999, the National Surgical Adjuvant Breast and Bowel Project (NSABP) selected 193 institutions to participate in its second major Breast Cancer Prevention Trial (BCPT). The STAR study (Study of Tamoxifen and Raloxifene), the largest breast cancer prevention trial ever conducted, is currently well underway. In this study, 19,000 postmenopausal women who are at above-average risk for breast cancer were randomly assigned to take either tamoxifen or raloxifene for 5 years. After that time, researchers will decide which drug most effectively prevented breast cancer with the fewest side effects. If raloxifene is effective in this trial, it will likely receive FDA approval as a breast cancer chemopreventative drug, giving women another option.

Women at high risk for breast cancer who are considering chemoprevention for this disease should ask their gynecologist about the present status of raloxifene and tamoxifen as breast cancer preventatives, based on results of the STAR trial (if currently available).

Prophylactic mastectomy Some women who test positive for

BRCA1 or -2 mutations may choose to have prophylactic mastectomy—preventive removal of the breasts. A study published in January 1999 in the *New England Journal of Medicine* revealed that prophylactic mastectomy may reduce the risk of breast cancer by 90 percent in women at high risk for the disease. Prophylactic mastectomy cannot reduce breast cancer risk by 100 percent, because it is not possible to remove all of the breast tissue.

This type of information, however, creates a conundrum for women found to have BRCA gene mutations. They are faced with the fact that surgery may greatly reduce their risk of developing breast cancer. On the other hand, the lifetime risk of breast cancer for women with BRCA gene mutations may be significantly lower than the 80 percent that was initially believed to be accurate. Therefore, while many women with BRCA gene mutations may save their lives by having a prophylactic bilateral mastectomy, others will choose this option even though they may never develop breast cancer.

Removal of ovaries and fallopian tubes: Since the ovaries are the major source of estrogen in a woman's body, and because estrogen plays a role in most (but not all) breast cancers, removing the ovaries and fallopian tubes (salpingo-oophorectomy) seems to decrease breast cancer risk by up to 50 percent in women with BRCA gene mutations. In addition, by removing the ovaries, the risk of developing ovarian cancer is greatly reduced. Risk is not eradicated completely, however, as sometimes small amounts of ovarian tissues are left behind.

Ovarian Cancer

Oral contraceptives: Though use of oral contraceptives (combined estrogen and progestin pills) reduces the risk of ovarian cancer in women at average risk, a recent study reported that Ashkenazi Jewish women with BRCA gene mutations did not experience a decreased risk of ovarian cancer with use of oral contraceptives. The conclusion of this study was that it is premature to recommend the use of combined oral contraceptives to women with BRCA gene mutations as a way to reduce the risk of developing ovarian cancer.

Transvaginal ultrasound and CA-125 measurement: Beginning at age 30, women with BRCA gene mutations should have an annual or semiannual screening, consisting of serum CA-125 measurement and transvaginal ultrasound (see CA-125 and TVU Tests for Ovarian Cancer, on page 164, for more information on these procedures). After the completion of childbearing, and by age 40, these women should consider having their ovaries and oviducts removed (see below).

Prophylactic salpingo-oophorectomy (preventative surgical removal of the ovaries and oviducts): A review of ovarian cancer prevention in the April 2003 issue of *Current Treatment Options in Oncology* concluded that the prophylactic surgical removal of both the ovaries and oviducts is the most effective method of risk reduction in women who have a high risk for ovarian cancer. As noted above, a salpingo-oophorectomy also decreases the risk of breast cancer in women with BRCA gene mutations, since it removes the major source of estrogen in the body. Therefore, this procedure may truly be the proverbial killing of two birds with one stone when it comes to lowering the risks of breast and ovarian cancers in women with BRCA gene mutations.

CAROTID ARTERY DISEASE TREATMENTS

Your therapy heavily depends on the extent of the disease. Ideally, arterial blockage will be discovered long before major surgical intervention is required. If this is the case, you can manage or even reverse carotid artery disease with medication and changes in your diet and lifestyle. If the blockage is far advanced, you have surgical options.

Lifestyle Management of Carotid Artery Disease

People whose carotid plaque buildup is not significant enough to warrant surgery should recognize that they have been given a life-saving wake-up call. Reducing all of the modifiable risk factors in your life is now essential to your future well-being.

Medical Management of Carotid Artery Disease

If you have significant but nonsurgical plaque buildup in your carotid artery, you should discuss statin (cholesterol-lowering) drugs and other medical treatments—like taking one baby aspirin a day—with your doctor.

Of course, you should also undergo diet and lifestyle changes to control your cholesterol. Several studies have now shown that effectively improving your lipid profile (lowering total and bad cholesterol levels and raising good cholesterol levels) can actually *reverse* plaque buildup on carotid arteries.

Surgical Management of Asymptomatic Carotid Artery Disease

There is no proven benefit to operating on a carotid artery that is more than 50 percent open. In that case, medical treatment is usually just as effective as surgery. If, however, your blockage is so severe (greater than 70 percent) that it requires surgery, there are two different common procedures.

Carotid endarterectomy: A carotid endarterectomy is a surgical procedure in which the carotid artery is exposed through an incision in the side of the neck. The major branch of the carotid coming into and going away from the area of narrowing is temporarily clamped, and the artery is opened. The atherosclerotic plaque that is causing the narrowing is then removed from the artery. The vessel is then sewn back together, and the clamps are removed. If a patient's blockage is greater than 70 to 80 percent in one or both carotids, recent data shows that this procedure can decrease the possibility of a future stroke by 50 percent.

As you might imagine, this procedure is not without risks. Because there is atherosclerosis in the carotid arteries, you may also have the same type of condition in your coronary arteries or other blood vessels. This increases the risk of a heart attack during the operation. It is also possible for nerves in the neck to be injured, causing weakness of your voice box, speech function, or tongue muscles. Furthermore, there is a possibility of a stroke during the operation or during the recovery period. In most major medical centers, the risk of stroke from this procedure is less than 3 percent. Carotid endarterectomy is also a relatively expensive procedure, with the total average cost for the diagnostic tests, surgical procedure, hospitalization and follow-up care averaging about $15,000.

Angioplasty: Angioplasty is a procedure that is being studied as an alternative to carotid endarterectomy. Balloon angioplasty with stent placement (like the procedure that is used in the heart arteries) is being tested. See "Coronary Heart Disease Available Treatments," on page 226, for a more detailed description of this procedure.

There is not enough data yet to know if this is a viable option to carotid endarterectomy. The most reliable data have found that carotid angioplasty can be performed with the same complication rate as carotid endarterectomy. However, it is too soon to tell if the long-term benefits are comparable.

COLON CANCER TREATMENTS

The purpose of having a colonoscopy when you have no symptoms of colon cancer is to avoid ever getting it, by finding the precancerous polyps that will eventually produce it.

However, for those people who are found to have an existing colorectal cancer after a colonoscopy, surgery and chemotherapy are the two most common options.

Surgery: Radical surgery is the only potentially curative therapy for colorectal cancer. When performed with the intent of cure, the primary tumor and the regional lymph nodes through which it could spread are removed. Patients who are found to have lymph nodes containing cancer cells are generally treated after surgery with adjuvant chemotherapy as well. The success of surgery in achieving a cure depends primarily on the stage of the cancer.

When all of the cancer cannot be removed, the surgeon removes as much of the tumor as possible to decrease symptoms, usually to prevent obstruction or bleeding. This is called palliative surgery. In some cases, palliative removal is not possible, and your doctor might then perform a bypass operation to prevent obstruction.

Chemotherapy: Chemotherapy drugs interfere with the production of cancer cells, resulting in cell death or the halting of tumor growth. Unlike radiation or surgery, chemotherapy is a systemic treatment (treating the whole body). It can reach cancer sites in the body that are not always accessible by other means. The goal of chemotherapy is to attack cancer cells with minimal side effects to the patient (although it is common to have some side effects).

Chemotherapy is given both to cure and to help control colorectal cancer when it cannot be cured. It is generally given to those patients whose tumors cannot be completely removed surgically and to those who may have undetected microscopic cancer cells remaining after surgery has removed all apparent signs of cancer.

CORONARY HEART DISEASE TREATMENTS

Lifestyle Changes and Medical Management

In general, patients whose coronary narrowings do not limit blood flow undergo lifestyle modification and receive medications to help prevent progression of CHD.

Lifestyle changes: These help prevent further buildup of fatty deposits in the coronary arteries. They are known to most people, and include quitting smoking, exercising regularly, reducing stress, controlling diabetes if you have it, managing blood pressure, and switching to a diet that lowers cholesterol and results in weight loss (if you are overweight). This last topic is very much in debate these days, and may mean switching to a diet very low in the simple carbohydrates that rapidly raise blood glucose levels, such as the South Beach Diet or Atkins Diet. These lifestyle changes are equally important for patients who also undergo more aggressive treatment, like angioplasty, stenting, or bypass surgery.

Medications: Many people with early CHD have angina (recurring pain or discomfort in the chest that happens when some part of the heart does not receive enough oxygen—it is a common symptom of CHD). Antianginal medications (such as beta-blockers, nitroglycerin, and calcium channel blockers) can reduce the symptoms of angina by reducing the amount of oxygen the heart requires. They also increase the amount of blood flow (and thus, oxygen) to the heart. Other medications include aspirin or aspirin-like drugs, cholesterol-lowering drugs, and agents that block the harmful effects of some hormones, such as angiotensin II.

Angioplasty and stenting: If a patient has limited blood flow in the coronary arteries, balloon angioplasty and stenting can be offered as treatments. Roughly one-third of patients with CHD will undergo these procedures. During balloon angioplasty, a balloon-tipped catheter pushes plaque back against the arterial wall to allow for improved blood flow in the artery. Another angioplasty technique involves devices that remove plaque from the arteries by cutting it away.

Coronary stenting often accompanies the angioplasty procedure. Stents are small wire-mesh metal tubes that provide scaffolding to support the damaged arterial wall, reducing the chance that the vessel will close again after angioplasty.

Coronary artery bypass surgery: In patients with multiple areas of coronary artery narrowing or blockage, coronary artery bypass graft surgery (CABG) is generally recommended. Of those patients found to have CHD, about 10 percent will undergo this surgery.

In a CABG, the surgeon uses a portion of a healthy vessel from the leg, chest, or arm to create a detour or bypass around the blocked portion of the coronary artery. CABG operations require general anesthesia and typically 4 to 7 days in the hospital. It may take up to 3 months to fully recover from the surgery.

ESOPHAGEAL CANCER
AND BARRETT'S ESOPHAGUS TREATMENTS

Negative for Dysplasia

EGD with biopsies: Patients diagnosed with Barrett's esophagus *without* evidence of dysplasia or esophageal cancer should have an esophagogastroduodenoscopy (EGD) with biopsies every 2 to 3 years and take action to decrease symptoms of GERD. This usually means eliminating acid reflux.

Diet changes: The most practical approach to eliminating acid reflux is through changes in diet. Avoiding foods like alcohol, tomato juice, orange juice, and foods high in caffeine or high in fat can reduce acid reflux. Elevating your head while sleeping can also help.

Medication: There are also several medications that can suppress the stomach's acid production and decrease reflux into the esophagus. A class of medications called proton pump inhibitors is commonly used to treat reflux in patients with Barrett's esophagus. Five different formulations of these drugs are currently available in the United States, and all of them are acceptable options.

Surgery: Patients who have severe GERD may be candidates for surgery designed to reduce reflux. Surgery, of course, is expensive and always entails some risk, so you should discuss this option thoroughly with your doctor before taking it.

Low-Grade Dysplasia

Repeat EGDs: Patients with Barrett's esophagus who have low-grade dysplasia should have repeat EGDs at 6 and 12 months, followed by annual EGDs if the lesion has not progressed. In addition, these patients should also take action to decrease symptoms of GERD (see the section above, "Negative for Dysplasia").

High-Grade Dysplasia

The finding of high-grade dysplasia in Barrett's may indicate that cancer of the esophagus is already present. Therefore, when high-grade dysplasia is found, the EGD should be repeated immediately and more biopsies taken.

Endoscopic ultrasound: Also, endoscopic ultrasound (EUS) may be used in patients found to have Barrett's with high-grade dysplasia. This technique can help determine if in fact cancer is present, and determine the depth and amount of tissue involved (see EUS and ERCP for Pancreatic Dysplasia or Cancer, on page 188, for more information on endoscopic ultrasound). Endoscopic ultrasound is almost always available in large hospitals that have doctors specializing in Barrett's esophagus or esophageal cancer.

Esophagectomy: This is the gold standard for management of high-grade dysplasia, but this is a major surgery. Esophagectomy involves removal of most of the esophagus, leaving a small amount at its upper end toward the mouth. The small segment of remaining esophagus may then be hooked to the stomach (by pulling the stomach up), or the surgically removed section of esophagus may be replaced with a segment of colon.

Patients with Barrett's or early adenocarcinoma who opt to undergo an esophagectomy should seek out an experienced surgeon with a good track record. This is extremely important, as all surgeons are not equal in skill. Even if you have to travel a long distance to a major medical center to get a good surgeon, it may be of great benefit in the long run. The death rate (mortality) associated with esophagectomy is near zero percent in most hospitals today. However, after the surgery, a number of complications may arise, including hoarseness, delayed emptying of the stomach, and narrowing of the gut due to scar tissue formation.

Photodynamic therapy: In the past few years, photodynamic therapy (PDT) has been used to treat patients with Barrett's esophagus with high-grade dysplasia or superficial esophageal cancer who are not good candidates for esophagectomy. The idea behind PDT is to kill the highly dysplastic cells of Barrett's esophagus before they become a true cancer (or before they spread, if they already have evolved into an early cancer cell). A November 2002 report in the *Mayo Clinic Proceedings* suggests that PDT is an effective treatment for the abnormal tissue found in Barrett's esophagus, as well as for superficial esophageal cancer. Their study involved 48 patients, 34 with Barrett's esophagus with high-grade dysplasia, and 14 with early esophageal adenocarcinoma. After just one course of PDT, the abnormal tissue and cancer cells were completely eliminated in 27 of the patients. Twenty of the 21 remaining patients underwent a follow-up PDT procedure, which eliminated the rest of the abnormal tissue.

Watchful waiting: Some patients with high-grade dysplasia in which cancer has been ruled out may opt to just have frequent follow-up EGDs. In these individuals, the EGD is done initially every 3 months for at least a year and then less frequently. How frequently will be determined by your doctor, but every 6 months or so is common after the first year if no changes are seen. This type of approach requires patient compliance (don't miss appointments!) and that the patient understands that there is no absolute guarantee that if you are in fact destined to get adenocarcinoma of the esophagus, it will be found in a curable stage. However, the odds are much stronger for a better outcome than if you had high-grade dysplasia and did nothing at all.

Esophageal Cancer

If a screening EGD determines that you already have esophageal cancer, the treatment you will be given will depend on the stage of the cancer. In general, there are three options.

Surgery: This is the most common treatment for cancer of the esophagus. The procedure is an esophagectomy, as described in the section above, "High-Grade Dysplasia."

Radiation: Radiation therapy is also used to treat esophageal cancer. This technique uses x-rays or other high-energy rays to kill cancer cells and shrink tumors. Radiation may come from a machine outside the body (external radiation therapy) or from putting materials that contain radiation through thin plastic tubes into the area where the cancer cells are found (internal radiation therapy).

Chemotherapy: Chemotherapy uses drugs to kill cancer cells. Chemotherapy with or without radiation is being tested in clinical trials. In addition to use as a long-term treatment after diagnosis, chemotherapy and radiation therapy may also be used before surgery in some patients who have esophageal cancer.

HEMOCHROMATOSIS TREATMENTS

Phlebotomy: People who are found to have hemochromatosis due to HHC or for nongenetic reasons can undergo phlebotomy (blood-letting), which lowers total body iron content. It is essentially the same procedure that people undergo voluntarily at the blood bank, except that patients with hemochromatosis usually need a large number of phlebotomies in a relatively short period (blood donors generally only give a pint every 56 days at most). Also, patients with hemochromatosis are depending on the treatment and cannot be sent away if the phlebotomist finds it difficult to find a vein and remove blood.

Diet and medication: In addition, patients are often placed on low-iron diets, or may use medications called chelaters to remove iron from the body. Also, as alcohol can significantly exacerbate iron overload disease, patients should limit their intake.

Early diagnosis of hemochromatosis is imperative, since it is one of the few diseases where a simple, effective therapy exists. If hemochromatosis is found and therapy begins before the onset of chronic disease, life expectancy is normal. By contrast, the late signs of hemochromatosis typically do not develop until a significant amount of iron has accumulated, usually in patients who are 40 to 60 years of age. By that time, these patients will have a reduced life expectancy, even with treatment.

HEPATITIS C TREATMENTS

Approximately 75 to 85 percent of people infected with HCV will develop a chronic, or long-term, infection (often present the rest of their lives). Of these, an estimated 70 percent will develop chronic liver disease. Around 15 percent or so of people who become infected with HCV fend off the virus themselves and never need treatment. The goal of treatment for HCV is to eliminate the virus from your body early to try to avoid progression to cirrhosis and serious, end-stage liver disease. Once end-stage liver disease has set in, the only treatment is a liver transplant.

Diet and medication Depending on the viral load and how early the disease is detected, many people remain healthy for a long time without medications, simply by completely abstaining from alcohol use and by eating a healthy diet. Following these protocols will help prevent damage to the remaining healthy liver cells.

Medical Management

Usually, doctors will analyze a small sample of liver tissue through a biopsy, and if the biopsy indicates cirrhosis (severe scarring of the liver), precirrhosis, or substantial inflammation of the liver, most doctors recommend beginning treatment. For people with normal biopsy results, medical treatment is not usually recommended, and the disease will be monitored closely.

Alpha interferon and ribavirin: At present, HCV is treated with alpha interferon, a protein made naturally by your body that boosts your immune system. Alpha interferon can either be used alone (monotherapy) or in combination with the antiviral drug ribavirin (combination therapy). Combination therapy is significantly more effective in reducing the HCV viral load to undetectable levels.

Vaccination: It is also recommended that people with HCV are vaccinated against hepatitis A and hepatitis B. Hepatitis C infection does not increase your chances of getting hepatitis A or hepatitis B, but having both infections at the same time may make an HCV infection worse.

People who are diagnosed with HCV may also want to visit the Web site of Naomi Judd, the country music star who was diagnosed with HCV in 1991 and forced to retire from her singing career. She was quite ill at the time, but underwent treatment and today is doing very well. She has a Web page regarding HCV and her personal story, which can be seen at www.focusonhepc.com/naomi1.html.

HIV-POSITIVE INDIVIDUALS—TREATMENTS

The decision to start medications is somewhat complicated. Your doctor will probably want to test your plasma viral load (PVL) several times a year to see if the amount of HIV in your blood is changing and may consider starting you on HIV medicines if your PVL is higher than 55,000 copies per milliliter of plasma (using RT-PCR testing). Your doctor also has to consider the other medicines you are taking and other health problems you might have.

Another way to help decide when to start medications for HIV infection is to take a look at the CD4+ (helper) T-lymphocyte cell count. The CD4+ cells are the primary targets that HIV attacks. Therefore, if the PVL test score goes up, the CD4+ cell count usually goes down. A high PVL count coupled with a low CD4+ count is sometimes the trigger your doctor needs to see before she will decide it is time for HIV medication therapy. There may also be benefits to starting HIV medication if you know you acquired the HIV infection within the prior 6 months.

Antiretroviral Therapy

Antiretroviral therapy is a name for treatment with drugs that help prevent HIV from reproducing and infecting cells in the body. Antiretroviral drug therapy is effective in reducing the level of circulating HIV in the blood, raising CD4+ T-cell counts, preventing the development of complications, and prolonging life. These benefits may last several years in some people. However, these drugs do not help everyone with HIV, and there remains uncertainty about how to make the best use of the available agents, especially as these drugs can cause other serious medical problems.

Most of the antiretrovirals are aimed at just two targets in the HIV's life cycle: proteins called proteases and reverse transcriptases.

There are three categories of antiretroviral drugs that are available by prescription or clinical trials that work in this manner.

Nucleoside reverse transcriptase inhibitors: NRTIs act by blocking a step in the reproduction of HIV called reverse transcription. This step is necessary for HIV to be prepared for incorporation into the genetic material of human cells.

Nonnucleoside reverse transcriptase inhibitors: Nonnucleoside agents (NNRTIs) also block HIV reverse transcription, but they do so in a different way than nucleoside drugs.

Protease inhibitors: PIs work by blocking the action of protease, a protein made by HIV, which the virus must have to reproduce and infect new cells.

Side Effects

Antiretroviral drugs, while life-saving for many people, may themselves may cause serious medical problems. Metabolic changes are occurring in people with chronic HIV infection. One of these changes causes HIV-associated lipodystrophy syndrome (HIV-LS). This condition results in abnormal fat distribution and cholesterol and glucose abnormalities. Gender and HIV infection itself can influence cell metabolism, making it difficult to distinguish adverse drug effects from the natural progression of the disease.

Some anti-HIV drugs are toxic to mitochondria, the energy producers in cells. Tissues that require high levels of energy, like muscles and nerves, are most susceptible to the affects of damaged mitochondria. A disrupted mitochondrial energy supply can result in muscle wasting, heart failure, peripheral nerve damage causing numbness and pain, low blood cell counts, swelling and fatty degeneration of the liver, and inflammation of the pancreas. Other more general signs include fatigue, depression, and high lactic acid levels in the blood.

Osteonecrosis, or weakened bones, is another condition that is being seen more frequently in persons with HIV infection that may be a side effect of anti-HIV drugs. Talk to your doctor about having a DEXA scan (see page 172) to evaluate your bone mineral density if you have been taking antiretroviral drugs for several years.

Fusion Inhibitors

Combination therapy: In March 2003, the Food and Drug Administration (FDA) announced the accelerated approval of Fuzeon (enfuvirtide) for use in combination with other anti-HIV medications to treat advanced HIV-1 infection in adults and children ages 6 years and older. Unlike the other classes of antiretrovirals used for HIV, fusion inhibitors actually prevent the entry of the HIV virus into cells, so that it cannot replicate itself.

As might be expected when a disease caused by an infectious agent such as a virus is treated chronically with drugs, drug resistance in the HIV virus is on the rise. Because antiretrovirals that are in the fusion-inhibitor class work very differently than protease and reverse transcriptase inhibitors, they will likely be very useful in the treatment of drug-resistant strains of HIV.

HNPCC TREATMENTS

If you are found to have a known MMR gene mutation leading to the diagnosis of HNPCC, you should have increased surveillance for the most common cancers that can occur in HNPCC patients.

Colon Cancer

This is the most common cancer that occurs in people who have HNPCC. For people who are found to carry one or more of the MMR gene mutations that cause HNPCC, there are at least three recommendations.

Colonoscopy surveillance: The United States Multisociety Task Force on Colorectal Cancer released guidelines in 2003 for colorectal cancer screening. The Task Force recommended that people with HNPCC should have a colonoscopy every 1 to 2 years beginning at age 20 to 25, or 10 years earlier than the youngest age of colon cancer diagnosis in the family—whichever comes first. This frequent screening is recommended in people with HNPCC because they tend to grow polyps that progress rapidly from a small size to cancer. The daily use of small doses of NSAIDS (such as aspirin or ibuprofen) as well as folic acid supplements may be useful in slightly decreasing overall risk of colon cancer in HNPCC patients.

MSI detection in stool: As noted in the chapter on HNPCC genetic tests, microsatellite instability (MSI) in tumor cells is associated with colorectal cancers that occur in patients with HNPCC. Thus, testing colorectal tumor cells for MSI is a way to determine if subsequent genetic testing is appropriate in patients who already have colorectal cancer and a piece of their tumor has been obtained.

Now there is a way to test for MSI in tumor cells in people who have not yet been diagnosed with colorectal cancer but meet the Amsterdam II family history criteria for possibly harboring an MMR gene mutation.

After a colon cancer begins to develop, it sheds tumor cells containing its DNA into the stool. A new product called PreGen-26 identifies MSI in the tumor's DNA in a stool sample. It is a safe, noninvasive technology designed to detect colorectal cancer early in patients with known or suspected HNPCC, but who do not yet have colorectal cancer.

Remember, PreGen-26 is *not* a predictive genetic test. It was designed only for early detection of *existing colon cancer* in HNPCC patients or suspected HNPCC patients. It is most effectively used in conjunction with frequent colonoscopy screenings. You should use PreGen-26 as a screening tool only after discussing it with your doctor.

Prophylactic removal of the colon: Surgical removal of the colon prior to a diagnosis of colorectal cancer is obviously the most drastic measure to prevent colorectal cancer in a known HNPCC patient, and such a decision can only be arrived at after discussions with your doctor and a qualified and experienced colorectal surgeon.

Ovarian Cancer

TVU and CA-125 testing: Women over 30 years of age carrying HPNCC gene mutations should schedule an annual transvaginal ovarian ultrasound combined with an annual CA-125 blood test (see CA-125 and TVU Tests for Ovarian Cancer, on page 164).

Ovariohysterectomy: After the childbearing years, it is recommended that women with HNPCC talk with a knowledgeable physician about the possibility of prophylactic removal of both ovaries and the uterus.

Uterine Cancer

Endometrial aspiration biopsy or ultrasound: Women with HPNCC gene mutations should have an endometrial aspiration biopsy or ultrasound annually after 30 years of age.

Ovariohysterectomy: As noted above for ovarian cancer risk, after childbearing years, it is recommended that women with HNPCC talk with a knowledgeable physician about ovariohysterectomy as a preventative procedure for these cancers.

Renal Pelvic and Ureter Cancer

Blood tests and urine cytology: In HNPCC families with at least one member having a urological cancer, testing for urinary blood every few months and urine cytology every 1 to 2 years starting at age 30 to 35 is recommended.

Stomach Cancer

EGD: In HNPCC families with at least one member having stomach cancer, EGD every 1 to 2 years starting between ages 30 and 35 is recommended (see page 180 for more information on stomach cancer testing with EGD).

Cancer of the Small Intestine

Upper GI series: In HNPCC families with at least one member having cancer of the small intestine, an upper GI series every 1 to 2 years starting at age 30 to 35 is recommended.

KIDNEY CANCER TREATMENTS

Surgery

This is the most common treatment for kidney cancer, even in its earliest stages.

Simple nephrectomy: This surgery removes the whole kidney. If the kidney on the other side of the body is healthy, it can take over filtering the blood.

Radical nephrectomy: This removes the kidney with the tissues around it, including some lymph nodes in the area. Partial nephrectomy removes the cancer and part of the affected kidney; this is usually done only in special cases when the other kidney is damaged or has already been removed.

Other Therapies

The therapies listed below are generally only employed if there is evidence that the cancer has spread beyond the kidney.

Chemotherapy: This therapy uses drugs to kill cancer cells that have spread throughout the body. Chemotherapy may be taken by pill, or it may be put into the body by injecting it into a vein.

Radiation therapy: This treatment uses x-rays or other high-energy rays to kill cancer cells and shrink tumors. Radiation may come from a machine outside the body (external radiation therapy) or be received by materials that contain radiation through thin plastic tubes inserted into the area where the cancer cells are found (internal radiation therapy).

Biological therapy: Biological therapy (also called immunotherapy) helps the body's natural ability (immune system) to fight cancer or protects the body from some of the side effects of cancer treatment. Monoclonal antibodies, interferon, and interleukin-2 are some types of biological therapy.

LUNG CANCER TREATMENTS

In all cases, the detection and treatment for lung cancer must be early in the disease process for an actual cure to be possible.

Thoracic surgery: Removing all or part of a lung is the most radical option for early lung cancer, and the one most likely to produce a cure if the cancer has not spread far. The type of surgery performed may be a wedge section (removes only a small part of the lung), a lobectomy (removal of an entire lobe of the lung), or a pneumonectomy (the removal of an entire lung). Some tumors are inoperable (cannot be removed by surgery) because of the size or location, and some patients cannot have surgery for other medical reasons.

Radiation therapy: Also called radiotherapy, radiation therapy involves the use of high-energy rays to kill cancer cells. It is directed specifically to the area where the tumor exists. Radiation therapy may be used before surgery to shrink a tumor or after surgery to destroy any cancer cells that remain in the treated area. Doctors also use radiation therapy combined with chemotherapy as a primary treatment instead of surgery.

Photodynamic therapy: Photodynamic therapy (PDT) is more than 90 percent effective in the treatment of certain types of early-stage lung cancer. A special light-activated drug is injected that accumulates in the tumor tissue. A low-energy laser light "switches on" the drug, which then destroys the tumor cells.

High–dose-rate brachytherapy: Known as the "smart bomb" of cancer treatments, HDR brachytherapy delivers high doses of radiation directly to the site of the tumor using a computer-guided radioactive pellet. Today's precise mapping capabilities make HDR brachytherapy an effective treatment option.

Chemotherapy: This option of destroying lung cancer cells by impeding their growth and reproduction is usually reserved for more advanced stages of lung cancer.

OSTEOPOROSIS PREVENTION AND TREATMENT

There is no cure for osteoporosis if it is diagnosed. But it is a manageable disease when found early, and is a highly preventable disease as well. If you catch it early (or simply are at high risk for it), there are many courses of action available to you to keep it from advancing. Each of the BMD assessment categories described in DEXA Scan for Osteoporosis, on page 172, has a different treatment plan.

Normal DEXA scan: A normal DEXA scan in someone at above-average risk for osteoporosis suggests that you have probably been doing the right things—you probably have a diet high in calcium and vitamin D, do regular weight-bearing exercise, don't smoke, and don't drink excessively. On the other hand, maybe you did none of these things and are just lucky.

Whatever the case, if you are at high risk for this disease, you must remain vigilant. You now have an accurate baseline DEXA T-score to work with. By changing your modifiable risk factors in a favorable direction and having another DEXA scan in 5 years to monitor your progress, you can greatly decrease your risk for acquiring this skeletal problem.

Osteopenic DEXA scan: If a DEXA scan shows you have osteopenia (low bone density that has not progressed to true osteoporosis), but you do not yet have any fractures, it is time to make some behavioral changes in your life. You should begin an exercise program that includes weight-bearing exercise of some type—even walking or jogging is helpful. Smoking, caffeine, and excessive alcohol use can accelerate bone loss, so if these are issues, you need to quit.

How aggressively you treat osteopenia also depends on your age, as the relationship between osteopenia and future fractures is highly correlated with age. If osteopenia is left untreated, the risk of a fracture will double with every decade past age 50. A young person with osteopenia does not have much risk of fracture, but if no prevention is done, the lifetime risk will be about 20 or 30 percent.

PREVENTING LOW BONE MASS

Hormone replacement therapy: Hormone replacement therapy (HRT) in postmenopausal women decreases the risk of developing osteoporosis and the fractures associated with it. However, as the overall risks of HRT may exceed its overall benefits, you should discuss traditional HRT with your gynecologist.

HRT in men: Men who have low testosterone levels should talk to their physicians about testosterone replacement therapy. This is especially true of men who have low testosterone levels and whose DEXA scan shows osteopenia.

Other medications to prevent osteoporosis: Currently, the FDA approves alendronate, raloxifene, and risedronate for both the prevention and treatment of postmenopausal osteoporosis. Other drugs can be used in both men and women who already have osteoporosis, but the above drugs are useful for preventing the onset of the disease.

Drugs can also be used to treat osteopenia. Estrogen improves the bone density more than drugs such as alendronate and calcitonin. However, as we have noted, the safety of HRT is currently in question. Therefore, deciding to use estrogen is something you need to work out with your doctor. Tamoxifen or raloxifene also have estrogenic effects in bone, and can be considered for use in people with osteopenia. See the section on breast and ovarian cancer on page 219 for more information about tamoxifen and raloxifene.

Osteoporotic and established osteoporosis DEXA scan: Although osteoporosis cannot be cured, it can be managed. As with osteopenia, one of the first things your doctor will advise is behavior modification, including exercise and reducing or eliminating

Exercise: If you are at risk for osteoporosis, get to the gym and start lifting weights moderately, or do stair climbing. Alternatively, start a walking or jogging regimen. All of these activities have been shown to be effective in preventing bone loss (in addition to the other benefits of exercise).

Calcium and Vitamin D supplementation: A daily calcium intake of 1,000 milligrams daily up to age 50 and 1,200 milligrams daily over age 50 is very helpful in preventing osteoporosis. However, keep in mind that calcium cannot be absorbed into your body effectively without an adequate amount of vitamin D in your body. Normally, we make enough vitamin D from exposure to as little as 10 minutes of sunlight a day. If exposure to sunlight is inadequate (which may be the case in winter), then vitamin D intake from supplements should be at least 400 IU, but not more than 800 IU per day. Most calcium supplements now come with vitamin D already added.

smoking, alcohol, and caffeine. In terms of drug therapy, calcium supplementation (to a total of 1,500 milligrams/day) in combination with vitamin D (400 IU) is always recommended. Estrogen replacement therapy or use of tamoxifen or raloxifene are also options that should be discussed with your doctor.

For preventing hip, vertebral, and wrist fractures, other drug treatments may help.

OVARIAN CANCER TREATMENTS

The nature of the treatment for ovarian cancer depends on a number of factors, including the type of ovarian cancer, the stage of the disease, and the general health of the patient. A team of specialists often treats patients, and may include a gynecologist, a gynecologic oncologist, a medical oncologist, and a radiation oncologist.

Surgery: This is the usual initial treatment for women diagnosed with ovarian cancer. The ovaries, the fallopian tubes, the uterus, and the cervix are usually removed. This operation is called a hysterectomy with bilateral salpingo-oophorectomy. To find out if the cancer has spread, the surgeon also removes lymph nodes and samples fluid from the abdomen and tissue from the diaphragm and other organs in the abdomen. If the cancer has spread, the surgeon usually removes as much of the cancer as possible in a procedure called tumor debulking. Tumor debulking reduces the amount of cancer that will have to be treated later with chemotherapy or radiation therapy.

Surgical side effects include short-term pain and tenderness in the area of the operation, which can be controlled with medications. For several days after surgery, the patient may have difficulty emptying her bladder and having bowel movements.

When both ovaries are removed, a woman loses her ability to become pregnant. Some women may experience feelings of loss that may make intimacy difficult. Also, removing the ovaries means that the body's natural source of estrogen and progesterone is lost, and menopause occurs soon after the surgery. Symptoms of menopause can be relieved with hormone replacement therapy; however, deciding whether to use HRT is a personal choice. Women with ovarian cancer should discuss the possible risks and benefits with their doctors.

Chemotherapy: This treatment may be given to destroy any cancerous cells that may remain in the body after surgery, to control tumor growth, or to relieve symptoms of the disease. Most drugs used to treat ovarian cancer are given by injection into a vein. There are, however, other methods. Some anticancer drugs are taken by mouth. When given intravenously or by mouth, the drugs enter the bloodstream and circulate throughout the body. The drugs can also be given through a thin tube, called a catheter, that is placed into a large vein and remains there as long as it is needed. Another method, called intraperitoneal chemotherapy, keeps most of the drug in the abdomen. In this procedure the drug is put directly into the abdomen through a catheter.

Regardless of the method used, second-look surgery may be performed to examine the abdomen directly after chemotherapy is finished. The surgeon may remove fluid and tissue samples to see whether the anticancer drugs have been successful.

Radiation therapy: Also called radiotherapy, radiation therapy involves the use of high-energy rays to kill cancer cells. Radiation therapy affects the cancer cells only in the treated area. The radiation may come from a machine (external radiation) or from a liquid that is put into the abdomen through a catheter. This treatment is called intraperitoneal radiation therapy.

Radiation therapy, like chemotherapy, affects normal as well as cancerous cells. Side effects of radiation therapy depend mainly on the treatment dose and the part of the body that is treated. Common side effects of radiation therapy to the abdomen are fatigue, loss of appetite, nausea, vomiting, urinary discomfort, diarrhea, and skin changes on the abdomen. Intraperitoneal radiation therapy may cause abdominal pain and bowel obstruction.

PANCREATIC CANCER TREATMENTS

Surgery: For pancreatic dysplasia and early (Stage I) pancreatic cancer, surgery is the most common treatment. Depending on the extent of the lesions or tumors, this surgery may be a partial pancreatectomy (the head of the pancreas, part of the small intestine, and some of the surrounding tissues are removed), a distal pancreatectomy (the body and tail of the pancreas are removed), or a total pancreatectomy (the entire pancreas and the organs around it are removed). Surgery is frequently followed by chemotherapy and radiation therapy.

Although removing the pancreas has significant medical downsides (complications from the surgery include problems digesting food and also diabetes, because the pancreas is our natural source of insulin), researchers conclude that removing the entire pancreas with its precancerous lesions outweighs the risks of surgery. Studies show that leaving *any* part of the pancreas behind in patients with pancreatic dysplasia results in a high incidence of pancreatic cancer within 2 to 10 years.

PROSTATE CANCER TREATMENTS

If you are found to have prostate cancer, the first thing your doctor will try to determine is whether your cancer is confined to the prostate (localized disease) or has spread (metastasized) to other tissues. Localized disease is potentially curable, and we discuss the treatment options below. Bear in mind that deciding on a treatment plan is not a simple process because the growth and mortality rates for prostate cancer vary widely and are dependent on a great number of factors.

Watchful waiting: Deciding to watch and wait after a diagnosis of prostate cancer is generally based on the patient's age and the grade of his prostate cancer. A number of well-conducted clinical studies have found that men with well-differentiated, localized prostate cancer have excellent long-term survival rates.

Radical prostatectomy: Since 1991, removal of the prostate, or radical prostatectomy (RP), has been the most common treatment for localized prostate cancer. It is the initial treatment for more than one-third of newly diagnosed patients, most commonly men under age 75. The procedure is usually performed with the intent of curing men who have a life expectancy of at least 10 years. Radical prostatectomy is generally followed by 3 days of rest in the hospital, then 3 to 5 weeks of rest at home.

After the prostate is removed, it is sent to the pathology department for further evaluation. The margins of the prostate are inspected for cancer cells. If they do not have cancer cells, it is assumed that the cancer was confined within the prostate and has not spread outside it. However, if they contain cancer cells, some prostate cancer cells may remain in the body, and further treatment, such as radiation or hormonal therapy, may be necessary.

Surgery to remove the prostate is not risk-free, of course. Since men who have a prostatectomy no longer produce semen, they have "dry" orgasms. There can be other, more serious complications as well. Prostatectomy may cause permanent impotence and can also lead to urinary incontinence, but these side effects are less common today than they were in the past. When this surgery is successful, impotence and urinary incontinence are only temporary.

Radiation therapy: Radiation therapy is the second most common treatment for prostate cancer and is the most common treatment for men between 70 and 80. There are two types of radiation therapy commonly used to treat prostate cancer.

EBRT: External beam radiation therapy (EBRT) may cure the cancer if it has not gone beyond the prostate gland but will only slow the growth of the cancer if it has already spread beyond the gland. EBRT uses a high-energy x-ray machine to direct radiation to the prostate tumor. The procedure lasts a few minutes at a time and is repeated 5 days a week over the course of 6 to 8 weeks. EBRT is an outpatient procedure, so it does not carry the standard risks or complications that accompany major surgery.

There are, however, many disadvantages to EBRT. The length of treatment—5 days a week for almost 2 months—can be inconvenient, particularly for people who do not live near a radiation treatment facility. Also, choosing radiation treatment over surgery provides no opportunity for your doctor to examine lymph nodes around the prostate—a step that can determine exactly how far the cancer has advanced.

There are also several short-term side effects associated with EBRT. Rectal irritation and diarrhea occur in 30 to 50 percent of patients. Bladder irritation occurs in about 30 percent of patients, causing frequent or urgent urination and sometimes a burning sensation when urinating. Fatigue may last for several weeks after treatment is completed. There can be temporary skin changes, including redness, dryness, scaling, and itchiness of the treated area.

Long-term adverse effects are also possible with EBRT. Erectile dysfunction can occur, developing gradually 2 to 5 years after treatment ends. The chance of erectile dysfunction after radiation therapy may be as high as 30 to 40 percent in men younger than 65, and 50 percent in men 65 and older.

Brachytherapy: In this procedure, radioactive seeds are placed directly in the prostate tissue. This technique was first developed in the 1970s but was abandoned shortly thereafter because of problems with inaccurate seed placement. Starting in 1983, use of the transrectal ultrasound probe improved the procedure, and there has been a resurgence in the practice. Brachytherapy is most often used alone for men with well- or moderately differentiated prostate cancer that has not metastasized, or in combination with EBRT for men with more aggressive cancer that has still not yet metastasized. Brachytherapy has a number of advantages, including the following:

- It is a convenient outpatient procedure, and typical patients can resume normal activities quickly.

- Since radioactive seeds are inserted directly into the prostate, it minimizes radiation exposure to surrounding tissues.

- Incontinence of urine occurs in only a small subset of patients, and impotence rates are less than with the other therapies.

- Ten-year results show that the vast majority of patients remain disease-free, making it an attractive alternative to both radical surgery and full-course EBRT.

Cryosurgery: Also referred to as cryotherapy or cryoablation, cryosurgery involves the freezing of the prostate gland in order to destroy it. Probes are inserted into the prostate and are then reduced to a very low temperature.

Prostate cryosurgery has been used since 1968 and has become increasingly popular as it has become more refined. While it is currently not a routine therapy, it will likely become more common for the treatment of cancer that is confined to the prostate.

STOMACH CANCER OR GASTRIC DYSPLASIA
TREATMENTS

Low-Grade Dysplasia

Low-grade dysplasia means that there are some atypical changes in stomach cells, but that these changes do not involve most of the cells, and the growth pattern of the glands is still normal.

Frequent monitoring with EGD: If low-grade dysplasia in the stomach is the finding of your biopsy taken during an esophagogastroduodenoscopy (EGD), you and your doctor will discuss a plan to use frequent monitoring with EGD to see if and how the problem develops—remember, there is an 80 to 95 percent chance these changes will *never* progress to stomach cancer in this instance, but they bear watching.

Vitamin C and beta carotene: Further, just as it is wise to eradicate *H. pylori* from your body *before* it leads to the premalignant changes in the stomach, it is also wise to eliminate this bacterium from your body if an EGD shows that you already have these premalignant changes, because these could cause additional cell changes leading to a true stomach cancer. There are some studies that show that if EGD is used to follow patients with premalignant changes, such as mild dysplasia, after eradicating *H. pylori*, the amount of premalignant change in the stomach declines. Nonetheless, at the present time it does not seem wise to completely avoid any follow-up EGD testing if you have mild (low-grade) dysplasia in the stomach simply because you eliminated the *H. pylori* infection.

There may be more you can do for yourself if you have premalignant changes in your stomach. A study reported in the December 6, 2000 issue of the *Journal of the National Cancer Institute* found that antibiotics, vitamin C, or beta-carotene—a precursor of vitamin A—can reverse precancerous stomach conditions.

In this study, researchers took stomach biopsies from about 1,200 migrant workers from the southwest part of Colombia. (Surveys had shown that these people were prone to getting stomach cancer at about five times the rate of other Colombians.) Of those whose biopsies showed abnormal cell growth in the stomach, some received a placebo pill, others received vitamin C (1 gram, twice daily) or beta-carotene supplement (30 milligrams, once daily), and still others received antibiotics against *H. pylori*. One final group received a combination of drugs and supplements. Those who were getting one or both of the supplements or the antibiotics were about *five times more likely* to experience regression of premalignant cell changes compared to those getting a placebo. It should be noted that none of the study participants with severe dysplasia (the last stage of stomach disease before cancer) improved significantly with any of the treatments.

Eradication of *H. pylori*: The vast majority of people with precancerous changes in stomach cells (or even stomach cancer itself) will have an existing *H. pylori* infection. Therefore, testing for the presence of *H. pylori* (and eradicating it if present) in patients found to have dysplastic changes in stomach cells should be part of the treatment of this disorder.

High-Grade Dysplasia

As with high-grade dysplasia in the esophagus, a high-grade dysplasia found in stomach cells presents a more serious problem than a finding of low-grade dysplasia.

High-grade dysplasia in the stomach is much more likely to convert to a stomach cancer at some point (and as with the esophagus, stomach cancer might even be already present) than low-grade dysplasia. Therefore, the intervention is often more drastic.

Some doctors will simply assume that this finding will certainly lead to stomach cancer, and will recommend doing a partial or total gastrectomy (see below), depending on the extent of the dysplasia. Alternatively, some doctors may elect to use photodynamic therapy (see "Esophageal Cancer and Barrett's Esophagus Treatments," on page 228), or even endoscopic mucosal resection in the treatment of high-grade dysplasia in the stomach. In an endoscopic mucosal resection, saline is injected between the layers of the wall of the stomach, creating a cushion and lifting and separating the innermost layer. The physician uses a special device fitted to the tip of the endoscope that suctions the tissue into a transparent cap, allowing the physician to snare and cut it. This technique is particularly useful in removing flat lesions in the stomach.

Stomach Cancer

Surgery: The most common treatment for cancer of the stomach is surgery. If the cancer is limited to a small part of the stomach, it can be totally removed along with that part of the stomach, using a procedure called a **partial gastrectomy**.

If the cancer is larger, a **total gastrectomy** may have to be carried out, which includes removing all of the stomach along with the lower part of the esophagus and sometimes the spleen. The esophagus is then joined directly to the first part of the small intestine (duodenum).

TYPE 2 DIABETES TREATMENT

The chronically high levels of glucose that are present in both diabetics and prediabetics are very harmful to your body if left untreated—something has to be done to bring the glucose levels back toward the normal range. Lifestyle changes are very helpful in this process and should be investigated first. If these are ineffective, then certain types of drugs can be used to lower blood glucose levels.

Diet: Both diabetics and prediabetics need to begin avoiding simple carbohydrates (like sugars) and highly processed carbohydrates (like white rice and bleached white bread) that are rapidly converted to glucose in the gut and absorbed into the body. Too much glucose is their problem—foods that quickly increase blood glucose levels only worsen matters. Diabetics need to eat more complex forms of carbohydrates, more fiber, and more fruits and vegetables. These are the very foods that may have prevented the development of diabetes or prediabetes in the first place (and can prevent prediabetes from becoming diabetes!). What specific diet is best for you will be determined by your doctor and a dietician.

Drugs: Medical treatment plans for newly diagnosed diabetics often give only lip service to the lifestyle changes that are required to control diabetes and usually are not realistic about the difficulties encountered by patients who attempt major changes in their lifestyles. After a brief or cursory attempt at lifestyle changes by the patient, the physician will often quickly give up on any chance of success and begin using prescription drugs like the sulfonylureas and thiazolidinediones to lower blood glucose levels in these diabetics. Unfortunately, these and other "hypoglycemic" drugs can result in numerous and serious side effects, both in the short term and long term. In addition, the evidence is not strong that taking oral hypoglycemic medications reduces the long-term complications of diabetes.

Therefore, the use of prescription medications to lower blood glucose levels in people with diabetes should be the choice of last resort. It should only be used in patients who have put in a serious effort with diet and exercise and have been unable to effectively lower their blood glucose levels. It can also be used in patients who are unable to exercise for physical reasons. If a glucose-lowering drug is taken as permission to postpone or forego important changes in lifestyle in a diabetic, then the prescription has done a great disservice.

Exercise: Dietary changes and exercise are very important in the treatment of both prediabetes and full-blown type 2 diabetes. Your goal, of course, is to prevent yourself from ever actually developing type 2 diabetes. Good news: The Diabetes Prevention Program (DPP), a major clinical trial sponsored by the National Institute of Diabetes and Digestive and Kidney Diseases, reported that dietary changes and exercise alone over a 3-year period sharply reduced the chances that a person with an impaired oral glucose tolerance test (suggesting prediabetes) would go on to develop full-blown type 2 diabetes.

A 2003 study published in the journal *Diabetes Care* by researchers at the world-renowned Joslin Diabetes Center has reinforced the findings of the DPP. This study found that obese adults (including diabetics, prediabetics, and nondiabetics) who lost just 7 percent of their body weight and performed moderate-intensity physical exercise for 6 months improved their major blood vessel function by approximately 80 percent. This is a very encouraging finding, since CHD, heart attack, or stroke are the leading causes of death in at least 75 percent of patients with diabetes. Get tested, and get moving!

"The important finding of this study is that a weight loss as low as 7 percent can improve or reverse the early abnormalities of blood vessels that lead to atherosclerosis and CHD and that obese people get equal clinical benefit from weight loss, whether they have diabetes, prediabetes, or have normal blood glucose levels," said Osama Hamdy, M.D., the lead author of the study.

INDEX